THE SIMPLE GUIDE TO FIVE ELEMENT ACUPUNCTURE

T0349808

by the same author

Keepers of the Soul
The Five Guardian Elements of Acupuncture
ISBN 978 1 84819 185 3
eISBN 978 0 85701 146 6

Patterns of Practice
Mastering the Art of Five Element Acupuncture
ISBN 978 1 84819 187 7
eISBN 978 0 85701 148 0

The Handbook of Five Element Practice
ISBN 978 1 84819 188 4
eISBN 978 0 85701 145 9

THE SIMPLE GUIDE TO

FIVE ELEMENT ACUPUNCTURE

NORA FRANGLEN

SINGING
DRAGON

LONDON AND PHILADELPHIA

This edition published in 2014
by Singing Dragon
an imprint of Jessica Kingsley Publishers
73 Collier Street
London N1 9BE, UK
and
400 Market Street, Suite 400
Philadelphia, PA 19106, USA

www.singingdragon.com

First edition published by Global Books Ltd, 2001
Second edition published by The School of Five Element Acupuncture, 2007

Library of Congress Cataloging in Publication Data
Franglen, Nora.
  The simple guide to five element acupuncture / Nora Franglen.
    pages cm
  Originally published as: The Simple Guide to Acupuncture : The Five Elements.
Global Books, Ltd, 2001.
  Includes index.
  ISBN 978-1-84819-186-0 (alk. paper)
  1. Acupuncture. I. Title.
  RM184.F5863 2014
  615.8'92--dc23

                                                    2013024591

British Library Cataloguing in Publication Data
A CIP catalogue record for this book is available from the British Library

ISBN 978 1 84819 186 0
eISBN 978 0 85701 147 3

Printed and bound in Great Britain

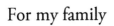
For my family

CONTENTS

About the Author

Nora Franglen has a degree in Modern Languages from Cambridge University, and worked as a translator whilst bringing up a young family. Her own experience of five element acupuncture led her to study at the College of Traditional Acupuncture, Leamington Spa, UK, and she continued her postgraduate studies there under J.R. Worsley. She was Founder/Principal of the School of Five Element Acupuncture (SOFEA) in London from 1995–2007 and continues her teaching through her practice, through postgraduate work in the UK, Europe and China, and now through her blog, norafranglen.blogspot.com. She lives in London, UK.

Preface

There are many branches of acupuncture, all of them basing themselves on the discovery in ancient China that needles inserted just below the skin into specific points on the body can help restore people to health. This book looks at acupuncture from the point of view of one particular branch known as five element acupuncture.

It has its own philosophical base, which is explained in the book, but uses the same routemap and seeks to achieve the same ends as any other branch.

The Chinese saw the elements as forces of nature whose energies pass through our bodies as organs. All illness is said to be the result of some imbalance in the relationship of the elements to one another, which places stress upon one or more organs. Treatment is directed at correcting this imbalance by inserting fine acupuncture needles into specific points which relate to the different organs.

What is exciting is that acupuncture can help restore a patient to balance by treating physical symptoms, such as headaches or a backache, as well as a patient's depression or ability to cope with stress. This makes it into a highly effective way of treating many of the illnesses which fill doctors' surgeries today.

The aim of this book is to introduce readers to this branch of acupuncture so that they can gain some understanding of the principles upon which it is based, appreciate through the case studies that are provided how beneficial it can be when applied, and then decide whether they wish to practise it or experience it for their own well-being.

CHAPTER 1

THE PHILOSOPHY UPON WHICH CHINESE MEDICINE IS BASED

According to Chinese philosophy, all things are manifestations of what is called the Dao. The Dao is the eternal, the infinite. It represents the universe before the Big Bang. All things, animate or inanimate, emerge from it for a lifetime to merge back again at their death. And everything reflects within itself an image of the original unity from which it has sprung.

For the world as we know it to emerge from the Dao, it has to break apart into two opposing and complementary forces, which the Chinese have called yin and yang.* Everything in the universe is created by this duality, which can be seen as the inside and outside of everything. It forms the pairing of all opposites:

---

* In Chinese, *yin* means the shady side and *yang* the sunny side of the mountain.

Hot/cold
Sun/moon
Night/day
Convex/concave
Black/white
Up/down
Inside/outside
Male/Female

Yin and yang, and their mutual interdependence, are depicted in the well-known symbol:

In turn, the pairing of yin and yang divides further into what are known as the five elements. The elements are seen as the processes of change and transformation which move the year from spring to summer and on to spring again, and move us from childhood to old age. In the human being they create the organs of our body. Heart, Stomach, Liver and Lungs* are all as much products of the work of the elements in our body as are spring and summer in nature outside.

---

* The Chinese regard the physical organs of the body as also incorporating an emotional aspect, indicated here by the use of capital letters (see pages 73–74).

(The five elements are explained more fully in Chapters 7, 17, 18, 19, 20 and 21.)

The Yellow Emperor and Acupuncture

Huang Ti speaks to Ch'I Po: I, who am chief of a great people and who should receive taxes from them, find myself afflicted by not being able to collect them because my people are sick. I desire, therefore, that the employment of remedies cease and that only the needles be used. I order that this method be transmitted to all future generations and that the laws concerning it be clearly defined, so that it will be easy to practise it, hard to forget it, and that it will not be abandoned in the future. Beside this, the actual modalities are to be accurately observed so that the way to research will be open.[*]

---

[*] From *The Yellow Emperor's Classic of Internal Medicine*. According to legend, the so-called Yellow Emperor is reputed to have lived in the 27th century BC.

CHAPTER 2

WHAT IS ACUPUNCTURE?

The word acupuncture means using a needle to puncture the skin. A fine needle is inserted just below the surface of the skin to stimulate points which lie along what are known as pathways of energy, called meridian pathways. These are distributed throughout the body, and can be seen as lines on a chart.

The human body is seen as a microcosm of the universe, a mini-world, with its seas and oceans, mountains and valleys. It has a surface, the skin, and depths beneath where the organs lie buried. The surface and the deep are connected by channels much as rivers flow deep within the earth to draw their waters from reservoirs within its bowels. At different intervals along these meridians there are places where needles are inserted, which are called acupuncture points.

For instance, a line joins the big toe to the eye, and the finger tip to the shoulder. There are small dots marked along each line and these dots are where acupuncture points are located. It is at these points that the needle is inserted.

The points used by acupuncturists today are the same as those used by acupuncturists working in medieval China, and, before that, in the China before the Christian era. This long history has meant that a great body of medical knowledge about the human being in health and ill-health has grown up over the centuries, providing evidence of acupuncture's effectiveness by its longevity and the sheer volume of documented case studies.

The meridian system which reaches every cell in the body can be likened to a central heating system in which the Heart is the pump, the different organs of the body its radiators and the meridians themselves the pipes along which the Heart pumps energy to all the organs and to every other part of the body. This network is like a more hidden version of the network of blood vessels. It is visible in places on the surface of the skin to a trained eye, and can be felt by a trained touch. It can be seen as channels of light by a technique called Kirlian photography.

Acupuncture is based on a view of the world very different from that which prevailed until recently in the West. It springs from a belief that man/woman and nature are one, part of a whole the Chinese call the Dao, the infinite. We remain healthy if we observe a state of balance with the natural world in which we live, which forms part of the Dao. We become ill if we disturb this state of balance in some way. Disturbance can be by external causes, such as pollution, drought or poverty, or by internal causes, such as an unhappy love-affair, bullying at school or discontent with work.

The aim of acupuncture is to use the needle to restore balance once more. The action of the needle adjusts the flow of energy through the meridian pathways, much as a plumber adjusts the flow of water through the central heating system. Unlike a hypodermic needle, the needles do not inject anything from outside into the body. They are used to stimulate the patient's own energy back to health.

It is considered good acupuncture practice to use the least number of interventions with the least number of needles to get the required result. It is therefore a method of least interference.

Illness can be seen as a patient losing control of their own health, and acupuncture treatment is aimed at putting them back in control. Acupuncture is therefore a form of natural healing. It encourages the patient's own energy to return to health and balance.

CHAPTER 3

HISTORY OF ACUPUNCTURE

To place acupuncture in its present context, you will need to know something of its history.

It originated in China several thousands of years ago, spreading from there throughout the Far East, before moving to the West. It appears to have arrived in Europe for the first time in about the 17th century. The first recorded case of acupuncture in England seems to be in 1827, when the writer describes acupuncture 'using a hat pin'. Acupuncture made its way to the United States from both Europe and the Orient.

Its history in China is very complex. It appears as a fully fledged medical discipline in written texts about the second century BC, and must have been in existence well before written records existed, probably as early as 1000 BC. There are even suggestions that stone needles were used, placing its origin far back in neolithic times.

Acupuncture has a history of continuous use from then to the present day, passing from country to country, from East to West, and in some senses also back again, in its travels. It has criss-crossed the globe much as the meridians of energy with which it works criss-cross the human body. It is the only system of medicine still in use today which has such a long and continuous history, and has travelled so far. It is truly tested by time.

Throughout the ages, individual masters of acupuncture developed their own styles of treatment, constantly adding new ideas to the body of knowledge built up in this way. Different schools of acupuncture developed as a result, and in turn gave way to other schools. As acupuncture travelled from country to country, and from continent to continent, with each transplanting it took on different characteristics.

Today there are numerous schools of acupuncture in many countries, East and West, all following their own traditions. They base themselves on the original Chinese texts, but with wide variations as to how these texts are interpreted, and with much new material which has been introduced over the centuries.

There are, therefore, numerous threads which together go to make up what we now band together under the name of acupuncture. Many traditions from many different Far Eastern, and now Western, countries form the body of knowledge upon which each individual acupuncturist bases his or her practice.

This book discusses acupuncture from the viewpoint of one of these branches: five element acupuncture.

Viewed from the long perspective of acupuncture in China, acupuncture's history in the West is so far very brief. It only emerged as an accepted system of medicine here after the Second World War, although a long tradition in France goes back a little further, as a result of France's contacts with Indo-China. Its time of true blossoming has been over the past 30 years or so.

A catalyst for the West's present interest in acupuncture was a visit by a *New York Times* reporter, James Reston, to China in 1971. He was given acupuncture to help the side-effects of surgery, and by writing about it ensured that acupuncture was brought to the attention of the Americans and of the world at large, and that its effectiveness became known to a much wider audience. Since then, the number of contacts between China and the West have grown enormously, leading to a corresponding increase in the West's interest in this peculiarly Chinese form of healing.

Paradoxically, the result of this burgeoning interest in acupuncture has been to rekindle China's own confidence in its home-grown system of medicine. The influx of Western medicine, first through the missionaries, and then through direct Western finance and encouragement, took place at a time when Western medicine, with its impressive arrays of life-saving drugs, appeared to be all-conquering. Against this tide, the voice of traditional Chinese medicine was temporarily silenced, only to come very much alive again, partly as a result of increased Western interest. The very high cost of Western medical interventions, which made it imperative for a developing country to find alternative forms of medical treatment, was one of the factors behind the renewal of interest in traditional forms of medicine in China.

As people in the West have become more aware of the risks of drug side-effects, this, too, has had the effect of turning attention to other, more natural forms of healing which do not involve such risks, among them acupuncture. All these factors have led to the phenomenal increase in interest here in the West. Whereas about ten years ago, people were surprised if you mentioned acupuncture, now there are very few people who have not heard of it, or who know somebody who has had it. Increasingly, people turn to it as stories of its success in treating different conditions abound.

Acupuncture has now found a firm foothold in mainstream medicine in the West. This has led to the present happy state of affairs, where it has become an acceptable form of therapy to the broad public, and increasingly to the Western medical profession itself.

CHAPTER 4

How Acupuncture is Used to Treat Illness

The acupuncture needle is the main instrument of treatment. Needles come in many shapes and sizes. A commonly used size of needle is shown here:

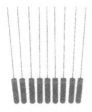

Acupuncture needles (approx. half actual size)

In the past, needles were made of gold, silver or bone, and what are thought to be stone needles have also been found. Nowadays they are made of stainless steel, and are always taken from a sterile pack for each patient and discarded after use.

The method of insertion and the needling techniques used vary according to the different acupuncture traditions. The needle can be used to stimulate the acupuncture point in different ways, and can be left in for varying lengths of time. Some acupuncturists give the needle a slight turn, before removing it immediately. In some cases, needles are left in the acupuncture point for some time if the diagnosis indicates a need for this. In others, the pulses will show that the needle needs to be inserted for a short time only. There is an accepted needle insertion depth for each point.

The needles are very fine indeed, very different from the thicker hypodermic needle we are familiar with from our visits to the doctor. Patients are often surprised and reassured to see how fine the needles are. When handled by a skilled practitioner, the patient does not feel the insertion of the needle into the skin, but there will, and should, be a sensation of some kind as the needle makes contact with the acupuncture point lying below the surface of the skin. This sensation can be anything from a dull ache to a sharp feeling, but it only lasts for a few seconds. There is little or no pain at all if the needle is left in the skin for some time.

The depth of insertion is not a guide as to whether the patient feels pain or not. Points on the surface of the skin may be more tender than those lying at a deeper level.

Treatment can be made more effective in certain cases by stimulating the point by heating a cone of a dried herb over it before inserting the needle. This technique is called moxibustion, the burning of moxa. Moxa is the Japanese for mugwort, a medicinal herb also well known in Western herbal medicine. The herb is dried and pulverized, and then formed into small cones which are placed on the acupuncture point and lit with a taper. It is removed when the patient says the cone has become warm. As with needling, there are many different ways of applying the herb.

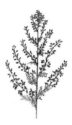

Mugwort

Each acupuncture point also lists the accepted maximum number of moxa cones which can be placed on it (for example, 3 or 11 cones). Moxibustion is a treatment in its own right, and may be used without needling on certain acupuncture points. It may be forbidden to use moxa in some cases, because adding heat to the point is not considered desirable (for example, if somebody has high blood pressure). It is excellent for people with low or normal blood pressure.

The needles and the moxa cones are used to stimulate the acupuncture points in such a way as to connect with the energy flowing along the meridians, and restore health and balance. How this is done will be discussed in greater detail in later chapters of this book.

The needles are inserted at different points for many different purposes. They can stimulate sluggish energy or calm down hyperactive energy. They can also increase the flow of energy through meridians that have become blocked, much like the waters of a dam can be released to irrigate parched lands further downstream.

They are not necessarily inserted near the site of pain, although they may be. Pain is a warning signal showing some disturbance of the smooth energy flow which indicates health. The cause of the pain may lie far away from the place at which we experience it, just as the land below a dam will suffer the worst drought, even though the water has dried up because it is dammed further upstream.

Let us take the example of a person with a headache. There are several meridians which pass over the head. If we follow the lines of the meridians, we will see that one starts on the hand and finishes at the nose, and another starts under the eye and finishes at the toes. If our diagnosis leads us to the decision that we should insert a needle in the first meridian, we might insert it at the hand to affect the energy running to the nose.

In the second case, we might insert the needle near the nose or at the feet.

We will see later on how and why an acupuncturist makes such choices of treatment. In both cases, we will hope to affect the headache, but in both cases, too, it is not the site of the pain which determines the treatment so much as the direction, flow and function of the meridians in the area of the pain.

Pain in the same place in two different people may be there for two different reasons and require two different treatments to clear it. We will discuss later on how we decide what treatment is needed in a particular case, and then how we decide where to insert the needle.

We will now look at how treatment can also be directed at helping people cope with symptoms that are not physical, such as the stresses of life.

CHAPTER 5

THE THREE LEVELS OF THE HUMAN BEING
Body, Mind and Spirit

It is important for an understanding of Chinese medicine that we look more closely at the different levels that exist within each human being.

We will use the example of the reader of this book. Your hands are holding the page and your eyes are scanning the words. Hands and eyes belong to your body, your physical part. Your mind then has to make some sense of the messages your eyes are sending to your brain. We call this the level of your mind. And finally when you start relating what is written here to your own experiences of life, particularly when what is mentioned touches on the personal or the emotional, you reach the deepest level, which is that of your emotions, your spirit.

If we listen to beautiful music, or watch the evening sky lit up by a wonderful sunset, that part of us which is stirred and moved by what we hear or see is our spirit. It is true that we first hear the sounds of the music physically, or catch sight of the evening sky with our eye physically at first, but a deeper response is woken within us.

The three levels of body, mind and spirit function happily together when we are in balance and healthy. Our bodies will move without trouble, our minds will think our thoughts easily and our emotional life will respond appropriately to the demands made upon it. It is when some stress occurs which overloads our capacity to maintain balance that problems occur. And this stress may occur at any level.

If we are studying for an exam, for example, we will overtax our minds. If we run a marathon, we will overexert our bodies. If we live in a dysfunctional family, we will damage our spirits. All three levels are inextricably linked, and we know this because our bodies cannot walk down the street leaving our minds working at the office desk.

The human being has a very complex body and inner life, capable of creating beautiful works of art and designing the most complex computer programmes. We do, however, have to pay a high price for our complexity. Just as racing cars break down more often than the simple tractor, so the highly evolved human being is more prone to illness than is a snail. One or other of the levels of which we are made can start to malfunction, putting further stress upon the other levels. If no help is forthcoming, all three levels start to show signs of distress and eventually there is total breakdown.

The sequence can be something like this: a man feels that his boss is unfairly victimizing him at work (stress at the mental level). He finds that he starts to get migraines on Sunday evenings as the worry of returning to work after the weekend swamps him (stress at a physical level added to stress at the mental level). As the weeks progress, the pressure gets worse. He can't sleep; he finds he's shouting at his children; he feels he can't cope at all (stress now moving to the level of the spirit, combined with mental and physical stress). He is hardly functioning at all. His boss sacks him on the grounds of incompetence, because his work has become erratic and his behaviour unbalanced. By now it is difficult to disentangle the level of his imbalance, since all three levels no longer function properly.

When this patient comes for acupuncture treatment, perhaps initially for help with a physical problem, such as the insomnia or the migraine, all the different levels of imbalance will be treated by inserting needles into parts of the body. The points also restore health and harmony at all the levels of the human being.

WHAT CAN
ACUPUNCTURE TREAT?

Most patients, when asked why they want acupuncture treatment, usually start with talking about physical symptoms, because they equate acupuncture with their understanding of Western medicine, which is that it treats physical problems. They are surprised when their acupuncturist asks them about their life in general, and shows interest in how they are coping with the stresses they are encountering.

As we saw in the last chapter, Chinese medicine does not regard the conditions from which people may suffer as falling into one category called physical and another called emotional. The human being is seen as one. If one part of us is in trouble, it will have a lesser or greater knock-on effect on the other parts. Chinese medicine also recognizes that constant stress from, for example, a divorce, can and usually does, have a big effect on a person's physical constitution, often making them more susceptible to disease. Equally, the physical effects of having severe migraines will make us feel emotionally ragged and unable to function at work as we should.

Since acupuncture recognizes the interconnectedness of the different levels of the human being, treatment is never focused on merely one level, but addresses wherever help is needed. Theoretically, therefore, there are no conditions, whether physical or emotional, that acupuncture cannot be used to treat, but in practice some conditions may prove resistant to help or have become so severe that they are beyond the reach of help. In such cases, acupuncture can often help alleviate, even if it cannot cure, and, in the case of the severely or terminally ill, it can help a patient cope better with what they have to face.

I would never say to a patient that I cannot help her, but I will always say that I will do my best and that I hope that she will feel some effects from treatment.

Because acupuncture can enable a person to cope with the stresses of life better, it is rare for a patient to feel absolutely no effects from treatment, but these effects can range from the complete removal of discomfort and pain to a feeling of greater well-being and ease or a temporary alleviation of pain.

There are many reasons why treatment may not prove effective. A patient may be too ill to benefit, or they may be exposed to constant stress, perhaps from heavy smoking or excess alcohol, which reduces or nullifies the effectiveness of any treatment. A healthy lifestyle, which includes such things as taking sufficient exercise, eating and drinking healthily, not staying up to all hours and resting when tired, will have a great effect on the success or otherwise of treatment. A patient's willingness to cooperate with the acupuncturist in improving his or her lifestyle is also a big contributory factor in whether or not they benefit from treatment.

How long does the treatment take?

The first encounter between practitioner and patient takes about two hours for a full diagnosis. At the next meeting, the patient will receive his first treatment, which may take up to a further two hours. After that, treatments last up to an hour each.

The speed at which patients feel the benefits of treatment varies. These can be gradual, as a person's energy is strengthened by each successive treatment, or there may be a quick response. A patient will report back on how they have felt in the intervening period, and the acupuncturist will base the next treatment on how the patient has felt, as well as on what the acupuncturist feels is required. To start with, treatment is at least once a week, for between eight and ten treatments. If somebody is very ill, they will benefit from more frequent treatments.

Once a patient starts to improve, and this improvement persists over a number of weeks, treatments will be spaced more widely, moving from once a week, to once in two weeks and then once a month and so on. Even when a patient's health is improving, they may choose to visit their acupuncturist when they find themselves subject to particular stresses at work or at home. They may also need particular treatments at the change of season, to enable their energy to adjust itself to changes in climate.

We can visualize the course of treatment in the following way:

Person out of balance   *After 3 treatments*   *After 10 or more treatments*

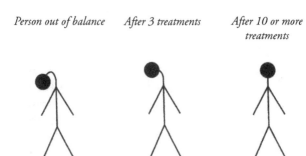

Each treatment brings a patient's energy more and more in balance, but it often has to struggle against old habits, which, as we know, die hard. We become set in our illness, much as we are set in our ways, and our energy has to be re-educated away from ill-health to the somewhat unfamiliar territory of health. This requires frequent treatment to start with.

The acupuncturist and the patient enter into a partnership for the period of the treatment. The acupuncturist, for his part, offers his skills to help move his patient towards health. The patient, for her part, accepts the need for punctuality and regular attendance, and must show a willingness to carry out any lifestyle changes agreed as necessary with the practitioner (such as reducing caffeine intake, eating regular meals).

The partnership is very close. The patient sees the same acupuncturist, and remains this acupuncturist's patient until she indicates that she wishes to transfer to another acupuncturist or until she stops treatment. The acupuncturist is there to help the patient make the necessary changes, and to support her while she is doing this.

Treatment requires work from both the acupuncturist and his patient. As we get better so things start changing, and a patient may find it a challenge to adapt to the changes required to benefit properly from the treatment. For instance, we may begin to see that our job or a relationship is hindering us from leading a happy life, and have to decide whether to change it and move on.

When we are out of balance, we may not be aware of where our greatest stress is, because everything stresses us. As we get better, so we begin to take a clearer view of what our life is about. This may lead us to see the need to change things. If, for example, we suffer from severe neck pain because we are lifting heavy loads at work, we may decide that it is time to change to a job which is less manual.

Acute insomnia: a case study

One of my patients had suffered from acute insomnia ever since starting work as a complaints manager for a telephone company. His treatment helped him recognize how much he hated dealing with people's anger. He asked for a transfer to another job in the company with less contact with irate customers.

Once he had made the decision to change his job, he began to sleep much better. In his case, treatment would not have helped him if he had continued in a job he found so very stressful, because any benefit from treatment was being cancelled out by the stress he encountered the next day. He had to decide whether he had the courage to look for another job, or whether he preferred the security of his present job despite the sleeplessness it induced.

We have to face choices such as these as we move along the path towards health. They are not easy to make, and we often prefer, somewhat weakly, to retreat into the familiar world of our imbalances rather than venture out into the apparently unknown. This is where the acupuncturist's close support is required to help a patient accept the need for change, and help him as he makes these changes.

CHAPTER 7

THE FIVE ELEMENTS

The five elements, or phases, are called Wood, Fire, Earth, Metal and Water.

These are words in common use and describe familiar aspects of life. We sit on wooden chairs when we sit on a park bench. We see fire whenever we light a candle. We dig up earth whenever we plant a bulb. We slice our bread with a metal knife. We slough off the day's dirt in water whenever we take a shower.

The elements symbolize the cycle of birth, growth, decline, death and rebirth to which all things are subject. Each element represents a stage along this cycle.

Wood is its beginning, its bud

Fire is its growth towards maturity, its blossom

Earth is its fruition, its harvest

Metal is the trace elements extracted from this harvest

Water is its moment of rest, as the new seed germinates

It is good that we should start our understanding of the elements with images drawn from the natural world: a bud, a harvest, a seed. Nature outside as we see it passing from season to season is a visible illustration of a cycle moving from element to element. We also see this cycle working in the rings a tree adds to its trunk each year.

These familiar words, with their practical relevance to everyday life, have been given meanings in Chinese philosophy which extend far beyond the everyday, and transform them into profound philosophical concepts. They encompass the processes given to the different stages of any cycle of activity, tracing their journey from start to finish. The different stages in the cycle of a day, a year and a lifetime are described in terms of the elements. The cycles of activity within our bodies which give us life and maintain us alive, and which in the West we know of as our organs, are also seen in terms of the elements. Symbolically, they represent all things in the process of change and development, and this includes our body as much as the year in nature outside.

In the West we have no overall philosophical concept which expresses cyclical activity of this kind, except as it appears in the individual seasons of the year and perhaps also the individual stages we pass through from life to death: birth, childhood, young adulthood, adulthood, maturity, old age and death (the so-called Seven Ages of Man).

To the Chinese, everything was subject to such phases of transformation and change, and this knowledge is used in their approach to health. The elements represent these different phases, and they shape the human being, making us who we are. They shape us physically, by creating the different organs of the body. They shape our bodies and our minds, and, as we shall see, they make us, by the unique interaction between them in us, the unique human being each one of us is.

An understanding of the cyclical activities underlying all things, and their relationship to different elements forms one of the fundamental tenets of traditional Chinese medicine. For us to understand health and ill-health from the Chinese point of view, we need to understand how the elements do their work within the different organs and functions of our body and how this work can be affected by the stresses placed upon us by life. We then need to understand how acupuncturists learn to diagnose the balance or imbalance of the elements in each of their patients, and to use the needle to correct any imbalances and restore health.

The sequence of the elements follows that of the seasons, as shown in the diagram on the next page.

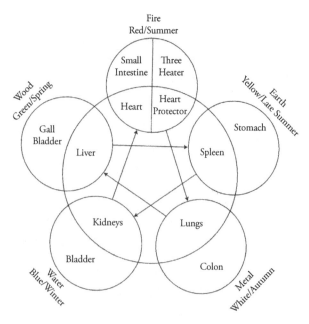

Each element is said to beget the next element, Wood being the mother of Fire, as Fire is the mother of Earth. Wood is also the child of Water, as Fire is the child of Wood. This is called the Law of Mother-Child in Chinese acupuncture. The cycle is a productive, beneficial cycle, as one element produces the next, just as one season produces the next season.

There is also another cycle, one of control, shown in the diagram by the straight lines across the circle. According to this cycle of control, Wood controls Earth (in nature you need roots in the earth to hold earth in place), as Fire controls Metal (metal needs to be tempered by fire if it is to be shaped), and Water controls Fire (water is needed if fire blazes out of control).

This control cycle can also turn destructive. Water can be harmful to Fire (a flood will put out the lights), or Earth to Water (silt damming up a river), or Metal to Wood (an axe cutting down a tree).

Each element is tempered by the others. None of them exists alone and its action is always modified and enhanced by that of the elements surrounding it. In a tight-knit family, which is that of the family of elements within us, none can work selfishly without damaging the others. Health is where an element is given the space to unfold as it needs to, whilst being supported by and supporting the other elements in their work. Ill-health is when one or other element concentrates so selfishly upon what it does that it has no time or desire to leave space for the others. It is as though the Heart were to work to the detriment of the Liver, or the Lungs to the detriment of the Kidney. Eventually the whole cycle of energy becomes unbalanced.

Serious illness and eventually death is the point at which all the elements are at war with one another. This would translate into a medical condition in which the Spleen starts to malfunction, the Kidneys fail and eventually the Heart fails as well. This, too, is how Western medicine regards the sequence of organ failure which precedes death.

CHAPTER 8

THE ASSOCIATIONS OR CORRESPONDENCES

The elements manifest themselves in many different ways. In nature, they are the different seasons of the year, with each element corresponding to a particular season. There are also numerous other areas of life, such as the time of day or a particular type of food, which the Chinese associated with the elements. They were fond of attributing symbolic importance to many things, and extended this concept of correspondences to include things such as the food we eat and the planets in the sky. (A very complex system of astrology is built up on these correspondences.)

Some of these associations, such as those relating to a particular season, are used diagnostically when treating a patient with acupuncture. Others have fallen into disuse over the centuries. The major associations used by acupuncturists today are the following:

- A time of the day

- Organs of the body

- Energy pathways (meridians)

- Acupuncture points along these meridians

- An emotion

- A colour on the skin

- A sound of the voice

- A smell on the body

The most important of these associations from the point of view of five element acupuncture are the last four: emotion, colour, sound and smell. The elements appear physically on our bodies, giving us a certain emotional imprint, a certain colouring to our skin, a certain tone to our voice and a certain smell to our body. These are very important indicators which acupuncturists use to assess a patient's state of health.

All of these diagnostic pointers can tell us something about our state of health. If the elements are in balance within us, they will express this by responding in a balanced way to the stresses of life upon them. They will adjust appropriately to the effects of the different seasons and different times of day. The organs they control will function appropriately. The energy flowing through the meridians they control will bring health to all parts of the body. The colours they impart to the skin and the sounds to the voice will be healthy indicators of their strength and balance.

Ill-health will show itself as the elements' inappropriate responses to such pressures. When an element starts showing distress, its associated emotion will show corresponding distress, so that a person's emotional responses begin to be inappropriate and erratic. We cry where we should laugh; we shout at our loved ones. The colours, sounds and smells that the elements project will also show that the elements are out of balance.

CHAPTER 9

THE GUARDIAN OR CONSTITUTIONAL ELEMENT

What makes five element acupuncture so fascinating is that it bases its diagnosis and treatment upon an understanding of what makes us the unique human being each one of us is. It sees this uniqueness as being created by a particular melding of the elements within us. This play of the elements in each one of us is the equivalent, in Chinese medicine, of what is known as our unique genetic imprint in Western medicine.

We can see this uniqueness in the fact that no Heart is shaped exactly like any other Heart, and no Liver exactly like any other Liver. So unique are we, that a single hair from our head or a drop of our blood can distinguish us so precisely from all the many millions of other human beings on this earth that it can trace a crime to our door.

Similarly, each human being has a unique elemental imprint, and one element, above all, takes up a dominant position. It is our constitutional element. I prefer to call it our guardian element. It gives us a certain approach to life, making some of us more serious and introspective, others more outgoing or vivacious. It spreads a certain hue over the colour of our skin, a certain smell on our bodies and a certain sound to our voice. It shapes our emotional responses, too, so that one of us is the sort of person who will view our troubles light-heartedly, whilst another person shaped by another element will be overwhelmed by the same troubles.

The qualities our constitutional element imparts to us have particular importance. Those with Wood as the constitutional element need structured movement and activity. Those with Fire need other people around them to relate to. Those with Earth need to nourish and sustain others and be nourished and sustained in turn. Those with Metal need to gain the respect of others and have quality in their lives. Those with Water need to feel secure. (See also Chapter 11 on diagnosis.)

There is much debate as to whether our constitutional element is something inherited or acquired, but it does seem as though the type of person we are is stamped upon us before we leave our mother's womb. A set of sextuplets seen on television showed between them the characteristics of all five constitutional types, and yet each had been born by Caesarian section within a few minutes of the others, and with no less or more trauma than any other of its siblings. Their mother described one as 'being always angry', the other as 'being the happy one' and yet another as 'the one who always looks after the others' – quite clearly differentiating between her children. We would have said that the first had Wood, the second Fire and the third Earth as their constitutional element.

In five element acupuncture, the constitutional element is the principal diagnostic tool by which we gauge a patient's health or ill-health.

Many other traditional systems of medicine use this concept of constitutional elements. A few centuries ago in England, this was known as the doctrine of the humours. According to all these systems of medicine, the elements or humours are regarded as creating specific human types. All are based on the belief that one of several constitutional factors within the human being is the cause of ill-health. In 17th-century England, your physician might diagnose you as being of the 'choleric' or 'phlegmatic' humour, and thus subject to choleric or phlegmatic types of diseases. In Chinese medicine, these humours are called elements.

Modern psychotherapy, too, recognizes different types of people, such as the introvert and the extrovert. Chinese and other forms of traditional medicine would regard these types as expressions of the elements. The ancient Greeks, the Indians, the Vietnamese, the Koreans, the Japanese, the Tibetans, all base their traditional forms of medicine on a similar understanding of this fundamental variety in the human being.

In constitutional medicine, the types of diseases and imbalances to which a person is subject will depend on the kind of person they are. Acupuncturists work on the understanding that you need to know the person before you can treat them. From such a perspective, people do not suffer from a common disease called high blood pressure. They suffer from a personal imbalance in their constitutional make-up which leads to high blood pressure.

If we are to treat the blood pressure, we must first discover the patient's constitutional make-up. The acupuncturist's function is to discover, not what disease a patient is suffering from, but who the patient is who is suffering the disease. Diagnosis, therefore, has a very different emphasis from that in Western medicine.

Treatment, too, will differ from patient to patient. One person with high blood pressure may be of one particular constitutional type, and require this particular series of treatments, whilst another with high blood pressure may be of quite a different constitutional type, and require correspondingly different treatments.

We each have a constitutional element, but the other elements which create our organs also play differing roles in our lives. They also colour the constitutional element, and are the means by which human variety reveals itself. We are the person we are and no other, because we are shaped by a unique combination of the elements within us. It is as though in one of us the Earth element is the most important element, but Wood is also important, but less so, and so on in diminishing order.

The yellow colour which the Earth element places on our skin will be tempered with a little green from the Wood element and lightened by a little white from the Metal element. In another person, their constitutional colour, red (Fire), may be modified by a little white from the Metal element and a little blue from the Water element. The other indicators, such as smell and emotion, will also be modified in this way. The joy of the Fire element can have a shading of sympathy within it if the Earth element is also there in strength. The anger of a Wood person may be hardened by the steel behind the Metal element within them, or softened by the warmth behind the Fire element within them.

CHAPTER 10

HOW AN ACUPUNCTURIST VIEWS HEALTH AND ILL-HEALTH

Living in Harmony with the Dao

The sense of connection with the Dao, the ultimate, which underlies all Chinese philosophy and Chinese medicine, implies that any disturbance of this connection brings ill-health in its wake. According to this philosophy, the aim of a healthy life is to learn to live in harmony with the forces of nature around us. Nature is seen as providing us with what we need to survive, and the belief is that nature, in its bounty, will have sufficient to satisfy all our needs.

This was no doubt true all those centuries ago in rural China, when a community could grow what it needed to live on. It is obviously less true nowadays, where pollution is rife, and global warming threatens fertile lands with floods and deserts; but there is nonetheless a great truth here which we need to take note of: we go against nature at our peril. We have seen this very clearly in the rising tide of man-induced problems, such as drug side-effects and the pollution of the air. It is as though we have cut ourselves off from our roots, and we all know what a plant's fate is if this happens. If we are not to wither, we must learn to re-connect ourselves to the natural world. We can do this by becoming more aware of the rhythms of nature, and one of the ways of doing this is to have acupuncture.

Whether we are able to remain healthy and thus in harmony with the Dao and the natural forces around us depends on many factors. Some of these are under our control; others are not. Yet others may have moved too far out of balance for us to help ourselves.

Some of those that are under our control are:

- Eating healthy, naturally grown food

- Eating foods that are in season

- Eating foods that are locally grown

- Drinking sufficient amounts of water

- Not drinking too much alcohol

- Not drinking too much tea or coffee

- Not taking recreational drugs

- Only taking prescription drugs where necessary

- Resting when we are tired

- Not over-exerting ourselves unnecessarily, either physically or mentally

- Learning to listen to the needs of our bodies

- Learning to avoid situations which stress us too much

- Learning to respond appropriately to the demands life makes upon us

- Learning to balance our own needs against those of the people around us

- Having the courage to change situations which stress us

- Finally: having the courage to assert our right to be ourselves, whilst not denying others a similar right

Some of those beyond our control are:

- Environmental factors

- Pollution

- Death

- The actions of other people

In acupuncture terms, we see the level of imbalance caused by overwhelming stress of any kind as an attack upon the healthy functioning of the elements within us. Their ability to respond to the demands made upon them has been impaired.

A person is considered to be healthy if all the elements are in balance with one another so that the organs and functions of the body are working in harmony. For example, if a person's Kidneys (Water element), Heart (Fire element), Lungs (Metal element) and Stomach (Earth element) function normally, we call that person in balance, and therefore healthy. Balance tilts to imbalance when one or other element and its associated organs ceases to function as it should. The smooth flow of energy from element to element becomes impeded at one point or other. This is what we call ill-health.

Once an element is in trouble, all the other elements band together to try and help it, like the members of a family rushing to the aid of a child in distress. In the early stages, before this distress becomes apparent in physical terms as pain or discomfort, it will already have shown itself to an experienced acupuncturist by the gradual appearance of signs of imbalance in the organs. We will see later that such signs can be seen physically on the body, and will be used diagnostically.

If continued stress over time has placed too great a pressure upon our ability to respond appropriately to any of the above, then we may no longer be able to cope by ourselves. This is when we have to turn to outside help to bring us back to balance.

There are many ways of doing things; we can go to a psychotherapist or a counsellor, or to our doctor. We can also turn to acupuncture.

CHAPTER 11

How an Acupuncturist Diagnoses

We have said that an acupuncturist has to discover who the patient is who has the disease or condition, rather than concentrating first and foremost on what disease or condition the patient has.

How do we go about doing this?
We need to find out as much as we can about our patients before we start treating them. We cannot decide on what the treatment should be until we have some understanding of how our patient approaches life, what their hopes and fears are, and what troubles they are coming to us for help with, whether physical or emotional. We have to give ourselves the opportunity to judge how the different elements are functioning in our patient, and which element is the dominant one.

All this takes time, and the initial encounter with our patient will take up to two hours.

What do we want to know about our patient? We need to know who she is, and what has happened in her life from earliest times to shape her as she is now. If she has come because she is distressed, what has distressed her, and when did this start? Why cannot she cope with this distress? Is it because it is a reminder of other pains long gone, but not yet laid to rest? Is her past life crippling how she is today? Is she in a relationship, and, if so, for how long, and is it a happy one?

What illnesses has she had in the past? What is she suffering from today? When did this start? What treatment is she having for it? If she is taking prescription drugs, what is the dose, and how long has she been taking them?

How has her health been from the day she was born (and sometimes even earlier if her mother had a difficult pregnancy, or she was an unwanted child)? Is the alcohol she drinks a habit over which she has control? Does she look after herself properly, feeding herself good meals? Does her appearance look cared for? Does she answer our questions openly, or is there much that is hidden behind a defensive screen? If so, how do we gain her confidence and trust?

But we do not just listen to the words. We listen to how the patient talks, and what she emphasizes as important. We listen to the sound of her voice, particularly when she touches on subjects which she finds emotionally disturbing, which is when the elements will show their presence most clearly.

We also look carefully at her as she talks. Which of the five element colours can we see? Does this colour change when she talks about something near to her Heart or disturbing to her? Is it a healthy or an unhealthy colour?

We try to detect the smell her body emits, particularly at times when what she is telling us is emotionally charged in any way, which is when the organs emit strong signals. If somebody suddenly starts talking angrily about their partner, we should smell a specific smell as the Wood organs express this anger.

And when we have gained this information, we go through a series of physical tests, including pulse taking, palpation of the body to assess any sensitive areas and assessment of body temperature. We look for any structural problems, like curvature of the spine, for any scars which might impede the flow of energy, for tightness of any muscles and we assess the condition of her nails and hair.

We also use this time of physical contact to assess our patient's response to touch, for this tells us much about her. Does she cling to our hand when we take her pulses, and is she therefore in need of support? Does she snatch her hand away, and is she therefore showing her vulnerability or anger?

Throughout this time we are continuously assessing the state of the different elements within her in many different ways.

Each element will show its imbalance in a different way. The first sign of trouble in the Earth element, for example, may be the appearance of an unhealthy tinge to the yellow of the face, or an exaggerated singing lilt to the voice. Maybe the patient finds she needs more support from other people than she usually does, craving attention where she is normally quite independent (Earth's emotion, sympathy, out of balance).

As an element becomes unbalanced it starts sending out signals of its distress. These signals come from the organs over which the element has control, and will appear physically in changes to colour, sound and smell, and changes to how a patient approaches life emotionally. Something happens over time to reduce its ability to cope. In the case of the Wood element, its organs – the Liver and Gall Bladder – send signals of distress to the surface of the skin. They cast a green sheen over the surface of the skin. They raise the voice to a shout, and emit a strong rancid smell. The person now reacts to situations with an anger out of all proportion to its cause.

These pointers all show Wood's imbalance, and will form part of an acupuncturist's diagnosis. For example, we know from Western medicine that our skin takes on a sickly yellowish-green colour when we become jaundiced. To a Western doctor, this is a sign that the Liver is diseased. In acupuncture terms, this is also a sign that the Liver (the Wood element) is in trouble, colouring the skin a sickly, not a healthy green. We would also diagnose the smell as being a sickly, not a healthy rancid, the voice as shouting and the emotion as inappropriate anger.

When a patient comes for treatment, therefore, the acupuncturist will be looking to see if the Wood element is in balance, or not. Does she plan and make decisions easily? Is any anger she shows appropriate? Is her colour green?

Is her Fire element in balance, or is she vulnerable to touch and afraid of relationships? Does her skin have the paleness we call lack of red, and is her voice unable to lift as she smiles?

Is her Earth element in balance? Is she capable of nurturing herself and others properly? Does she look after her diet? Is she able to process thoughts properly, or do they churn around in her head? Is her smell an unbalanced fragrant? Or her colour an unhealthy yellow?

Is her Metal element in balance? Has she been able to let things of the past go which are no longer appropriate for her, her previous relationships, perhaps, or the anger at her parents? Is she troubled by constipation? Has she breathing troubles?

Is her Water element in balance? Is she throwing up a front of confident behaviour behind which we sense uncertainty and fear? Has she a lot of willpower? Is her colour a healthy or unhealthy bluish-black? Does her voice hesitate, or is it a monotonous murmur?

Finally, we have to draw all these observations together, and make an assessment as to which element is the dominant, constitutional element.

We should get some of the answers to some of our questions during this first encounter with our patient. It will take much longer for both of us, patient and practitioner, to settle into each other and for our relationship to blossom. And this relationship is crucial to the outcome of treatment, for if we do not deeply understand our patient, and feel for her troubles, we will be unable really to 'see' her. She will elude us, and she may sense this and feel uneasy. If we are insensitive to her needs, we may well misinterpret or overlook the signals, both emotional and physical, which she is giving out.

Diagnosis continues as long as the patient comes for treatment, for she will come back for the next treatment a little changed by the treatment before, and, we hope, a little more herself, a little more in tune with what she needs to do and be. Each time we see her, we have to look at her afresh, as though diagnosing afresh, to see the state of the individual elements within her, and to assess what effect the last treatment had. This ongoing diagnosis forms the basis of each successive treatment.

CHAPTER 12

THE ASSOCIATION OF EACH ELEMENT WITH A SEASON OF THE YEAR

One of the simplest ways of understanding the elements is to see them in their most everyday and visible form – in nature, where they appear as the seasons of the year.

Wood is the season of spring

Fire is the season of summer

Earth is the season of late summer, harvest time

Metal is the season of autumn

Water is the season of winter

A closer look at the different qualities of each season will help us understand the qualities of the corresponding elements better.

The seasons will have a direct effect upon our health, for the balance of the elements in nature outside directly affects the balance of the elements inside each one of us. The changes nature undergoes as it moves through the year mirror what happens in the human being.

And what happens in nature outside affects each one of us. We may think that central heating and air conditioning protect us from the influences of the outside world, but experiments have shown that the blood in our veins rises and falls with the moon, whether we are enclosed behind walls or standing in the open. The sun's rays warming the earth will call forth a response from that part of us which belongs to the Fire element. The icy blasts of winter will evoke a response from our Water element.

We expect each season to have certain characteristics by which we recognize that all is well in nature. A summer which is hot, but not too hot, and drier than spring or autumn, but not too dry, gives buds a chance to unfold into full bloom. A summer which is cool or too wet will prevent the buds from developing to the full, or will drown the crops in the fields. If summer does not bring its expected gifts, nature will suffer, as the harvest withers on bough and stalk.

One of the questions acupuncturists ask their patients is what season of the year they feel most at ease in, and which they dislike. The answers patients give are very significant. They indicate a surprising variety in each person's experience of seasonal changes, with one person dreading the autumn and another being relieved when the hot summer days are over.

Little attention is paid in the West to these differences* but they are highly significant to acupuncturists. If a patient finds winter difficult, but revels in spring, this tells us something about the state of both the Water and the Wood elements within that person. It is also important to find out whether patients' seasonal preferences have changed. If a patient tells you that they find themselves more and more reluctant to go out in the sun, then we have to ask whether that person's Fire element (relating to summer) is in trouble.

Here there is a direct correlation between a patient's reaction to the changing seasons and the state of their health. When in balance, the elements should adjust to seasonal changes appropriately, so that we can enjoy the differing qualities of each season equally. Our Water element should enable us to enjoy the cold in winter, and our Fire element the heat in summer. If we dread either winter or summer, this shows that there is some problem in the Water or Fire elements within us. Any marked aversion is a warning sign, and the time of its onset must be pinpointed to find out what may have led to this change. This will form part of an acupuncture diagnosis.

When such preferences and dislikes started is significant, and we need to find out what was going

---

* Although a syndrome called Seasonal Affective Disorder is now recognized by Western medicine. This is nothing new to acupuncturists, who have always understood that feeling unwell in a season is a direct response by the elements to seasonal changes outside.

on in a patient's life at that time. Something which puts stress on the Water or the Fire element must have occurred to make a patient unable to tolerate cold or heat where before they could. As we will see later on, the stresses which lead to these imbalances can be emotional as well as physical. We may have lost our job or a loved one, or lived for a year in Finland. The change in either emotional or physical climate has affected our capacity to cope with heat or cold.

CHAPTER 13

The Chinese Pulses

Pulse-taking is a very important diagnostic technique in Chinese medicine, but pulses are taken in a very different way from those taken by Western-trained medical staff. Although the fingers are placed on the radial artery at the wrist in the same way, different pulses are felt at different positions along the artery. These pulses relate to the different organs. There are also two levels at which the pulses are palpated, one superficial and one deep.

On each wrist there are six pulses, making a total of 12 pulses in all, six at the superficial level of the wrist and six at the deeper level.

The middle three fingers are placed very lightly on each individual pulse position when we wish to take the pulses at the superficial level. They are pressed down slightly more to find the deep pulses below. For example, the Small Intestine pulse can be felt on our patient's left wrist with the index finger of our right hand. If we press a little more, we feel the Heart pulse just below it.

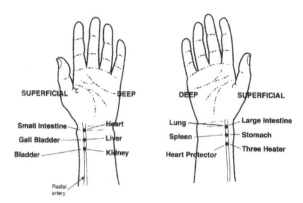

Pulses can also be taken elsewhere on the body wherever there is a strong surface beat, such as on the carotid artery on the neck, and on the tibial artery on the foot.

The art of taking the pulses according to the Chinese tradition is very subtle, and requires many years of practice to master. Students of acupuncture have to take a great many pulses each year of their training before really beginning to record accurately what these pulses are telling them. To the experienced acupuncturist, the pulses will reveal the state of health of the individual organs, through the signals that they send via the bloodstream to the surface of the body. An acupuncturist can discover the weak state of the Heart or the strength of the Colon from a reading of the pulses at the wrist.

Pulse readings will also record changes after acupuncture treatment, in many cases immediately afterwards.

The individual pulses will register different strengths and weaknesses and will show differences in pulse quality. Pulses are taken when the patient first arrives for treatment to provide information at the start of treatment, and will then be taken at regular intervals throughout treatment. How the individual organs respond to treatment will be noted, and used to plan the next treatment.

A pulse reading provides a great deal of diagnostic information about a patient's state of health, and will provide constant confirmation of the changes treatment brings about.

CHAPTER 14

THE CHINESE CLOCK
Law of Midday-Midnight

As well as imparting a specific quality to a different season, each element also has a relationship with a particular time of day.

We can understand this better if we think of the circle of the elements as a complete cycle of activity. This cycle continues within the cycle of one day, so that there is one part of the day which is associated with the Wood element, another with the Earth element.

Each pair of organs within the element shares a four-hour slot in the 24-hour cycle. The two pairs of Fire organs and functions share two four-hour slots. This means that the energy of each organ is at its highest at this time, and at its lowest at the corresponding time at the opposite part of the day or night. For example, the Stomach and Spleen are most active between 07:00 and 11:00 (by the sun), and least active between 19:00 and 23:00. The Lung and Colon are most active between 03:00 and 07:00, and least active between 15:00 and 19:00.

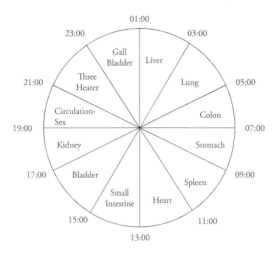

*These are times by the sun, and do not
take account of any daylight saving*

This is called the Law of Midday-Midnight, and is used to diagnose the balance of the elements within a patient. It is therefore very significant if a patient tells us that they wake up with a jolt at 01:00 (the start of Liver time), and cannot go to sleep again until 03:00 (the end of Liver time and the start of Lung time).

The function of the Liver (Wood element) in Chinese medicine is to make plans. Has the patient got problems with something she is trying to plan at the moment? Is that why she is waking up at this time? Is she trying to work out when it would be right to decorate the house, or have a holiday? Is this preying on her mind so much that the Liver starts to struggle at its time of greatest strength, waking her up in its struggles? She is only able to settle back to sleep again when the clock moves to the next part of the cycle, the Lung's two-hour period at 03:00.

Similarly, if somebody has digestive problems, and feels bloated after eating or craves sweet things, it may be because he is eating at the wrong time of the day. If he eats a heavy meal between 19:00 and 23:00, at a time when the Stomach and Spleen, Earth, are lowest in energy, he will not be able to digest the food properly, and it will lie heavy in his Stomach. According to the Chinese clock, we will digest our food best if we eat between 07:00 and 11:00, and best of all between 07:00 and 09:00 (Stomach time), to allow time for the Spleen (09:00–11:00) to pass the digested food on to the rest of the body.

If we have a healthy Earth element, it probably will not matter too much if we eat a heavy meal at night, because we are remarkably adaptable when we are healthy, and can cope with all sorts of stresses which overwhelm us when we are not well. If our Earth element and its organs are struggling for whatever reason, such as malnutrition, or an overprotective or needy mother who cannot nourish us (see Chapter 19 on the Earth element), our Stomach and Spleen's ability to take in food and digest it will be diminished. These organs will need all the help they can get from their period of greatest activity, which is 07:00–11:00.

A patient would then be advised to cook themselves healthy, nutritious food before 09:00, and have a much lighter meal in the evening, to try and help the Earth organs do their job at a time when they have the energy to do so, whilst avoiding stressing them too much at a time when they are at their weakest.

We have a saying which illustrates that it is not only the Chinese who knew this: 'Breakfast like a king, lunch like a prince and dine like a pauper.'

This Law of Midday-Midnight has all sorts of implications for the health of people working difficult hours, such as night workers, or people rushing to catch a train at 07:00, snatching a sandwich at lunch, and then spending their evenings eating heavy meals in a restaurant to recover from the day.

It also helps explain why so many people die in the early hours of the morning (03:00–05:00 Lung time), as the Lung 'breathes its last'.

It helps explain why most of us flag after lunch, as we move into Water's time (15:00–19:00). This is the time when we call upon our reserves (the Water element) to see us through the remainder of the day, and if these are low because we are tired, have not taken a proper lunch break, or have not nourished ourselves properly at breakfast, the time which should be our time of greatest energy boost becomes instead a time when we are drained of energy.

Anybody who teaches classes, as I do, knows to their cost that the most difficult time to keep students' attention is the late afternoon. A good glass of water (to feed their Bladder and Kidney) helps to revive the class wonderfully!

CHAPTER 15

THE ASSOCIATION OF EACH ELEMENT WITH AN ORGAN OF THE BODY

The elements create the individual organs of the body.

Wood	Liver Gall Bladder
Fire[*]	Heart Small Intestine
Earth	Stomach Spleen
Metal	Lung Colon/Large Intestine
Water	Kidney Bladder

You can see from this list that two organs belong to each element. For example, the Liver and the Gall

---

[*] The Fire element also has two additional functions, which are not related to an organ: the one known as Heart Protector, or Circulation-Sex, and the other known as the Three Heater or Thermostat (see Chapter 18 on the Fire Element).

Bladder belong to the Wood element, and the Lung and the Colon to the Metal element.

According to Chinese philosophy, the functions of the organs are more than just physical. They also function at the deeper levels, those of the mind and the spirit, which we have touched on before. We recognize these connections in everyday language when we say someone is heartbroken. We do not really think someone's Heart has broken physically in two, but we all understand what is meant by the phrase. The connection of emotion (love) to Heart is taken for granted, and is common to us all. We may not know where our physical Heart is, except perhaps somewhat vaguely in our chest, but we certainly know how our emotional Heart is functioning when we are happily or unhappily in love.

We also say that somebody has had the *gall* to say something to us (Gall Bladder), or that we cannot *stomach* something. When we are in an unhappy relationship, we may say 'I feel stifled by her', or 'He won't let me breathe' (the Lung). We also see other parts of the body in a similar way. Somebody is a 'pain in the neck', or we have a 'knee-jerk reaction'.

These examples from common speech show that we think of our body with its physical parts as more than just the body. The Chinese, too, saw that the individual organs had clearly defined connections with our deeper nature.

In Chinese medicine, each organ has a specific mental and emotional function as well as its familiar physical function. The Stomach, for example, processes our thoughts as well as our food. The Liver detoxifies harmful substances and plans the way we organize our life. The Colon gets rid of waste food products and of negative thoughts.

We will look at each organ's function in detail in the chapters on the individual elements.

CHAPTER 16

How the Elements Show Themselves in Us
Emotion, Colour, Sound and Smell

We will now look in greater detail at each of the principal diagnostic indicators of whether a person is in balance or not: their emotion, their colour, their sound of voice and their smell. As the elements become unbalanced, they start to send out signals of their distress, and these signals will appear as changes in our emotion, our colour, our sound of voice and our smell.

Emotion

We have seen that each element is associated with a different emotional response to life:

Wood relates to anger

Fire relates to joy

Earth relates to sympathy

Metal relates to grief

Water relates to fear

The way in which we respond emotionally will show the state of the elements within us. For example, when we show the emotion sympathy (the Earth element), an acupuncturist would say that our Earth element is in balance if the sympathy we show, and the sympathy we demand of others, is appropriate for the situation we find ourselves in. We show or demand neither too much nor too little sympathy. If we fall down, we do not expect the whole world to crowd round and help us (an excessive need for sympathy), nor do we reject expressions of other people's sympathy unnecessarily (an inability to accept sympathy).

But if our Earth element is out of balance, we respond inappropriately when sympathy is demanded of us, replying in a hard voice, 'I don't know what you're fussing about' if somebody asks us for support. An equally inappropriate response would be the over-solicitous, 'Oh, you poor dear!' to somebody who is coping well and in no need of such sympathy.

We think it normal if somebody speaks with joy of their children. We think it normal if somebody mourns a loved one deeply. We are disturbed by the apparent callousness of a person who shows no emotion when his father dies.

All the elements can express their associated emotion appropriately and inappropriately in this way. If we respond appropriately, we are showing that that particular element is balanced within us; if inappropriately, then there are problems of some kind affecting the element. For example, the person showing no emotion at the death of a father is a sign of lack of grief (Metal). There may be grief there, indeed it may be overwhelming, but it is being kept hidden and in check for some reason (perhaps fear of showing vulnerability or hidden anger). The grief which the Metal element is there to show is suppressed, a sign that this element is out of balance.

One of the first signs of trouble may be that a person starts to get irritated unnecessarily when the situation does not warrant anger. They may snap back at us when we ask a question (the Wood element's anger starting to show imbalance). If the Fire element becomes unbalanced, a person may giggle a lot (excessive joy). A person might laugh when talking about their serious illness (a sign of inappropriate joy), or sound sad when they are talking about their children (inappropriate grief).

We will discuss other examples of the emotions in and out of balance when we look at the individual elements in detail.

Colour

The organs also imprint themselves on the skin, again showing whether they are in balance or not. This colour has nothing to do with racial colour, and is as visible on somebody with a darker skin as a light skin. It is a hue spread over the whole body, but showing most clearly on the temples and around the mouth.

The Wood element imparts green to our skin

The Fire element imparts red to our skin

The Earth element imparts yellow to our skin

The Metal element imparts white to our skin

The Water element imparts blue to our skin

The colours may be healthy colours, showing that the elements in question are in balance, or unhealthy, showing that there is some problem. An example of a colour in balance is when we flush red with happiness. A sign of imbalance would be if somebody is very pale because they are anaemic or yellow because they have jaundice.

Sound

Our voices, too, express the elements' state of health:

Wood's voice is shouting

Fire's voice is laughing

Earth's voice is singing

Metal's voice is weeping

Water's voice is groaning

We can use our sense of hearing to gauge whether a person's voice is an appropriate or inappropriate expression of how they are, or whether it is expressing something quite different: groaning (Water) where laughing (Fire) would be appropriate, or singing (Earth) where shouting (Wood) would be appropriate.

If we are sensitive to others' needs, we respond to the emotional signals people's voices send us without being aware of it, smiling when we hear a laughing voice, and becoming quieter when we hear a weeping voice. If we are trained to do so, we will also hear the fear lurking behind the laughter, as we will hear the anger behind the sympathy. This will direct us towards problems in the Water element, disguised by the Fire element, in the first case, or problems in the Wood element, disguised by the Earth element.

Smell

The elements also emit certain smells which indicate whether they are functioning well or not.

The smell of Wood is called a rancid smell

The smell of Fire is called a scorched smell

The smell of Earth is called a fragrant smell

The smell of Metal is called a rotten smell

The smell of Water is called a putrid smell

These are the names conventionally given to the five different smells. Rancid, which is Wood's smell, is the smell of fresh vegetation when it is in balance, but moves towards the rancid when it is out of balance. Rotten is the lovely smell of fallen leaves on the forest floor in autumn when Metal is in balance, but the overpowering smell of rotting vegetation when it is out of balance. Putrid is a sharp smell when Water is in balance, but becomes the smell of stale urine (Water houses the Bladder and Kidney) when it is out of balance.

If we wish to diagnose the state of health of the elements within a patient, we have to learn to assess whether a person's body has the healthy smell which that element emits. For instance, if the element Fire is in balance there will be a warm scorched smell, but this smell will be too scorched if the patient's Fire element is overheating and burning them up.

All the elements have healthy colours, healthy smells, healthy tones of voice and healthy expressions of emotions. And then there are unhealthy, unbalanced manifestations of all these. In days long gone, a Western-trained doctor used similar skills to an acupuncturist, diagnosing what illness a patient was suffering from by the sick patient's smell. He would be able to tell whether a patient had tuberculosis, for example, by the smell in the sick room. Even now, a surprising amount of medical diagnosis is carried out initially by an experienced physician's observation of how a patient looks and feels.

We respond, often without being aware of it, to all the many signals we are sending out to each other in this way. Some of us will be attracted to a person's voice, others to the way they respond to us emotionally. Yet others, though we often are unaware of it, attract us by their smell. This is, after all, the secret behind the use of perfume. Different perfumes enhance a person's natural smell.

All these many pointers we are picking up unconsciously are regarded by acupuncturists as evidence of the workings of the elements within us. We are trained to trace these signals to their source, which we see as the action of the elements within each one of us.

This detective work is done by honing our senses. Acupuncture students need to learn to use senses often dulled by years of neglect. Animals and babies recognize people by their smell, and react instinctively in the presence of people they are uneasy with. The demands of civilized behaviour have tended to suppress these natural reactions (children are, after all, told they must be polite to everybody, even when their instinct tells them to avoid a certain person). Gradually, these instinctive reactions we are born with become atrophied, and we stop listening to their warnings.

A trained acupuncturist re-learns skills long unused, starts to use his eyes and his nose and his ears to pinpoint whether or not the signals the elements are sending show a balanced state of health or not, and then to direct him to where treatment is needed. In most cases treatment is seen in terms of the needs of the constitutional element.

As acupuncturists we use our senses to help teach ourselves how to distinguish the healthy from the unhealthy. We learn to gauge the degree of imbalance (ill-health) in a patient, and use what our senses have told us to decide what treatment our patient needs.

CHAPTER 17

THE WOOD ELEMENT

Season	Spring
Time of day	23:00–03:00
Climate	Wind
Organs	Liver Gall Bladder
Emotion	Anger
Colour	Green
Sound	Shouting
Smell	Rancid
Controls	Ligaments and tendons

There is no better place to start our journey round the elements than with the Wood element – its season, spring, representing the birth of a new year.

Spring is a time of new beginnings and new challenges. It is when we move out from the darkness of winter (the yin part of the year) into the light (towards the yang part). We can feel the renewed vitality in the air, as the days lengthen and become warmer. There is a vigour and force in the spring air, as life stirs awake after its winter sleep. Buds force their way out, with strength enough to break through concrete as they climb towards the light.

Hope is in the air. All things feel possible, as the future opens up before us. We feel invigorated. There is a bounce to our step, and a vigour to our thoughts. It is a time to get on and do things. We fling open the windows after months closed against the winter cold and spring-clean our houses.

Our bodies, too, benefit from the Wood element's energy, for it feeds the organs of our Liver and Gall Bladder. It also controls our ligaments and tendons, which enable the body to move, tightening and extending them to enable us to lift arm or leg, to turn our head, to stand up or sit down.

Every organ of the body has a specific function in Chinese medicine which extends beyond that of its known physical function. In the case of the Wood element, its two organs, the Liver and Gall Bladder, are involved in planning and decision-making.

Wood also has a lot to do with our eyes, and thus with vision in every sense, both physical vision (taking things in with our eyes), and mental vision (having the foresight to plan ahead).

Every movement we make requires planning. Even the act of lifting one foot in front of the other to walk requires commands to be sent to and from the brain to tell the tendons to tighten in such a way that the foot can be lifted, and then further commands to tell the same tendons to relax so that the foot can be placed on the ground in front.

The plan to lift the foot and the actual lifting of the foot (the decision to put the plan into effect) are under the control of the two Wood officials, the Liver and the Gall Bladder.

How do we go about planning a holiday, for example? We have to decide when and where to go. We have to work out an itinerary. We have to book flights and hotel rooms. When we sit down to plan the holiday, it is our Liver that does the planning sending off for holiday brochures, spreading out the maps, looking at available dates in our diary. When all this planning is done, the Gall Bladder takes over and makes the decision to book rooms in a certain hotel in a certain resort on a certain date.

The activities of the two are very interlinked. You cannot plan without making a few decisions about your plan, and you cannot decide without thinking about the plans, but the Liver can be thought of as the person sitting at home with the timetables and the Gall Bladder as the person talking to the travel agent, booking the flights and going to the airport.

Everything we do, from getting dressed in the morning to eating a meal and talking to a friend involves these two organs. We have to plan what words to say (Liver) and then decide to say them (Gall Bladder). We have to plan what clothes to wear (Liver) and decide to walk to the wardrobe to get them (Gall Bladder).

It is interesting to note that in Western medicine, too, the Liver is the busiest organ of all, involved in multiple planning tasks, such as metabolism of fat, detoxification of drugs, breaking down of carbohydrates and producing heat for the body.

When the Wood element functions well within us, it functions so smoothly that we are not aware that we are making plans and taking decisions. We just look at various options, decide on one and pick up the phone to book the holiday. When any organ is in balance, we will be almost unaware of what it does, like an engine that runs smoothly. It is only when a car starts to malfunction that we hear the gears grinding and the brakes squeaking. Similarly, our Liver and Gall Bladder can grind and squeak if they are not in balance.

Such signs of malfunctioning may appear as indecisiveness – one minute saying we will go to France, and the next saying we want to go to Florida (bad decision-making). Or we will write out a list of what we want to take with us on holiday, but forget to put suntan lotion on it (bad planning).

How does this element appear in a person whose constitutional element is Wood? Above all, these are people who need to have the room to move, but move to a plan. Buds, though about to burst out from their tight shell, burst open exuberantly, but in a structured way. The plan of the oak tree is there within the acorn, and the plan of the rosebush within the rosebud, before either unfurls into leaf and flower. Without that plan the buds would merely shoot out in all directions, and neither oak tree nor rosebush would grow.

Similarly, a person whose constitutional element is Wood (a Wood person) will need to keep his natural energy and vitality in check if he is to lead a productive life. He must move in one direction, forwards, not to left or right, for Wood is the element of the future. A plan has to be devised and a decision taken and acted upon. This is Wood's strength. In balance it will make excellent organizers, and do well in jobs where planning and decision-making are paramount. It will be quick at making these decisions, and they will be based on good judgement. It will speak and move energetically, and be happier striding out in the open than confined to a desk.

In its desire to get things moving, it will not suffer fools gladly (its emotion is, appropriately, anger), and be impatient if others do not move as quickly and decisively as it does. It will have a tendency to want to control others and shape them to its own plans. It needs space to unfold, and may push others aside if they stand in the way of its own expansion. It will respond to well-defined situations with clear boundaries within which it can expand to a set plan. It feels comfortable with structures which allow room for its own plans to develop.

It is also happy to set out the structures and boundaries for other people, giving the impression that it likes being in control, both 'I know where I'm going' and 'This is where you should be going.' Its strengths come to the fore when it is in balance and its organs are functioning healthily within us.

Now let's look at Wood out of balance. When life denies its buds the space to unfold or hinders its ability to structure what it does properly, its buds may remain partially unfurled. The plans it lays down now are incomplete. It loses the vision to see where it's going, or never develops such vision in the first place. Then all the gifts Wood brings become tainted, turning its blessings into curses.

Its desire for structure may become hardened so that it encases its life in boundaries which are too narrow and within which it gives itself no room to move. Its limbs may become arthritic, as the tendons and ligaments over which it has control lose their flexibility. It may confine its life rather than letting it unfurl freely. Its jaw may tighten with suppressed anger. Its plans may go awry because they are not well-laid. It may lose the ability to make any decision, or make them badly (suddenly giving in notice at work in anger without having planned what to do next).

Physically, its imbalance will show in an unbalanced green colour on the skin, a voice which may be either strident or drop to a whisper (inability to be angry), and a smell which becomes a sickly rancid. Its emotional responses may turn its natural impatience into blustery outbursts of anger. It may shout at people in an attempt to control situations over which it feels it has lost control, thinking the only way to do so is by raising its voice.

The Wood element: a case study

A man of about 60 came to me for treatment for help with very tight tendons in his legs. He found it difficult to bend his knees. As part of the diagnosis, he told me that he had been involved in numerous accidents, 'more than 15', he said, and at various times had broken bones in both legs and ankles, strained his back badly, and had had to be hospitalized with bad concussion three times. In all these accidents he had been the driver.

I diagnosed him as being of the Wood element. We have seen that the Wood element is all about movement forward, and is in control of our ligaments and tendons. It has a strong association with the eyes, and vision in every sense. We know it as the element which deals with planning and decision-making. We use our ligaments and tendons to move our limbs and our eyes to see where we are going, but to do this we have to have planned where we intend to go, and make the decision to get on and move.

When the Wood element is balanced, it will make an accurate assessment of the braking distance and time needed (good vision and planning), and then turn the wheel or apply the brakes at an appropriate time and with the appropriate amount of force to stop in time (good decision-making). The sight of an obstacle in front of the car is translated into the decision to slow down. In this patient of mine, however, we see the Wood element in trouble.

Instead of placing my patient in control of his car, his unbalanced Wood element made him lose control. He could not see trouble ahead in time, could not plan when to slow down in time and could not then put his foot on the brakes in time. All this meant that on many occasions he simply ran into the car in front, swerved suddenly or jammed on his brakes so that the car behind ran into him.

Nor did he appear to learn from his experiences. When I asked him whether he had ever wondered whether any of the accidents were his fault, he said angrily (Wood's emotion, anger, expressing itself inappropriately), 'No, I'm an excellent driver, though I say so myself. It's all these other bad drivers around.'

The vision which the Wood element gives us should have enabled him to see what was ahead of him, take avoiding action and ultimately understand the implications of his actions, if these actions result time and again in an accident. Like some child blaming the wall it runs into for its bruises, my patient expressed anger at what he could only see as the irresponsibility of others, being unable to see clearly both his car's position on the road and his own culpability in the accidents he was involved in. It was as though he was a child saying, 'You made me do it', blaming others, and sometimes his own car ('The brakes seemed sluggish') for his own driving errors. He appeared to learn nothing from each accident.

I also discovered that he was drinking heavily. We know from Western medicine that drinking affects the Liver, and will eventually lead to cirrhosis of the Liver and other serious problems. We also know that the Liver is controlled by the Wood element. The alcohol which affects Liver function, therefore, stops the Wood element from functioning properly. With each drink it loses more and more of its capacity to see what is ahead, to plan properly and to make the correct decisions. We see this quite clearly when we watch a drunk person veering erratically as they walk and falling over (the ligaments and tendons unable to hold the person upright).

My patient's treatment was not helping him whilst he was drinking away any effect it was having. I told him I could not treat him until he acknowledged that there was a problem, and took steps to stop drinking. To his credit, he listened and went away to think, returning some months later after having gone for help to an addiction clinic. He now no longer drank any alcohol.

Treatment consisted in strengthening his Liver and Gall Bladder officials. This helped improve the flexibility of his ligaments and tendons. The effects of treatment were quickly noticeable. He became aware that he was moving more easily. His walking was not so laboured, and he could bend his knees with increasingly less pain. The biggest effect, however, was on his sense of well-being. He said he had never felt better in his life.

He has been accident-free for the past four years. This would suggest that his Wood element now has sufficient ability to see what is needed, plan what to do and decide when to do it.

CHAPTER 18

THE FIRE ELEMENT

Season	Summer
Time of day	11:00–15:00 19:00–23:00
Climate	Heat
Organs	Heart Small Intestine
Functions*	Heart Protector Three Heater
Emotion	Joy
Colour	Red
Sound	Laughing
Smell	Scorched
Controls	Arteries

Wood is the 'get up and go' element, the part of each one of us that ensures that we get on with doing things. It is so engrossed in action that to some extent this

---

* The Fire element is the only element to have two associated functions as well as two organs.

makes it selfish. And this is right, for if a bud is to grow and develop, it can only do this by concentrating on itself.

But there has to be a part of ourselves which develops itself in different ways. One of these is through relationships. We need to turn to others, for we cannot live alone, otherwise the human race would die out.

That part of us which seeks others as friends or partners, and enables us to work in harmony with others in an office or workplace is the Fire element, the element of relationship.

Its two organs are the Heart and the Small Intestine. We all know what 'affairs of the heart' are, or have blamed someone for being 'heartless'. We seem to understand by this that the Heart has to do with relationships, above all sexual relationships. This, too, is how the Chinese saw the Heart within its element Fire. It pumps our emotional blood to help us maintain our emotional life, as it pumps our physical blood around the body to maintain life.

There must be warmth in our relationships to encourage them to grow and blossom, as the sun in the heavens encourages the buds of spring to grow and blossom. The Wood element requires the warmth of the Fire element to bring all its activities to bloom.

The summer, the time when the sun is at its height in the heavens, is when the Fire element, in us as well as nature, is at its greatest strength. We fling off our clothes in summer to greet the warmth of the sun. The world outside with its people beckons. Nature, too, flings wide its arms, as the trees unfurl to their greatest height, and all growing things reach their maturity.

Everything takes place in the open in the summer, as the warmth of the sun drives us outside. Windows stay open in the houses. We eat outside. We entertain our friends outside. We party outside. The life we lead is open to the gaze.

In a similar way, the Fire element lives its life in the open. When we relate to others, we have to reveal who we are to them. Some people reveal a lot about themselves, others prefer to keep some part of themselves well hidden. But we all have to show something of ourselves, and such exposure brings with it risks. We become vulnerable to what others can do to us if we lay ourselves open in this way.

The physical Heart, too, is a vulnerable organ, despite its importance to us, for we die the moment it stops to beat. To protect itself, it is hidden behind the ribs and encased in a muscular sheath, called the pericardium, but it is vulnerable to a single dagger's thrust between the ribs, which can bring death in its wake.

As we know, the Chinese viewed each organ as having deeper emotional functions as well. The pericardium is seen in Chinese medicine as something that protects the Heart not only physically, but also emotionally. At an emotional level, it protects the Heart from devastating emotional damage, the 'broken heart' we have all heard of. Its function is to ensure that the Heart is not damaged too badly in the first place, and, if damaged, is not damaged so irrevocably that a person is too injured to enter into any other relationship. The Heart Protector is the Heart's first line of defence, a protective wall thrown around it emotionally, much as the muscle of the pericardium is thrown around it physically.

Its capacity to protect the Heart depends upon how healthy and balanced it is. All the organs and functions have to be given time to develop themselves to the full. A young baby's Stomach, for example, has to learn how to process food slowly, relying first only on mother's milk, then on processed food and finally on unprocessed food when it has developed sufficiently to process such food itself.

All the organs grow slowly to maturity in this way. The Wood organs, for example, require time to teach the tendons and ligaments how to hold a young baby sufficiently firmly enough upright for it to sit, crawl, stand and finally walk.

Equally, the child's Heart and its Heart Protector need time to develop. A child will love indiscriminately from the moment it comes into this world, smiling on all with equal warmth. Only gradually does it become aware that some people are less friendly and others even dangerous. The people around a young child will help it develop its capacity to cope emotionally as well as physically, and, in the case of the Heart, develop its capacity to love appropriately.

In this way, its Heart Protector function will develop and mature slowly, helped by what we hope is wise advice and support from those around it. A parent or teacher, for example, will warn a child not to get into a car with a stranger. Similarly, young people may ask the adults around them for advice during their first sexual encounters to help them assess what is happening and make the right decisions. Young people also observe how others behave, and all this helps them develop their own protective mechanisms to support the Heart and ensure that the relationships they enter into do not harm them and are as balanced as possible.

Involved in all this are also the two areas of the Fire element we have not so far discussed, its second organ, the Small Intestine, and a further function called the Three Heater, or the body's temperature mechanism.

The Small Intestine in Western medicine is the organ which takes what the Stomach has processed, sifts it further, sending the good nutrients to the blood to be carried to the Heart, and the waste products to the Large Intestine or Colon for elimination from the body. Chinese medicine recognizes this physical function, and adds to it the further layers. We have to sift our thoughts, and only take on those which are useful, whilst discarding the others. We also have to sift our emotions, again passing only those judged to be good to the Heart, and discarding the others. This is the Small Intestine's work at all levels.

In physical terms, if the Small Intestine is not functioning properly, it will sift good from harmful products badly, passing the wrong material to the Heart, thus polluting the blood. The same can be true emotionally. This would be like somebody advising the Heart that this person was a most suitable person to have as a friend, whilst in fact they are trying to sell us drugs. If our Small Intestine is in balance, it would warn us against such an unwise friendship, rather than encouraging us towards it.

The final function is that of the body's thermostat, the Three Heater. It is called the Three Heater because in Chinese medicine the organs of the body are divided into three groups relating to three different areas of the body, and the relative temperature of the group of organs in each area is diagnostically important. The Three Heater keeps us physically as well as emotionally at an even temperature, neither too cold nor too hot. Physically, it helps regulate the temperature of the blood, and with it body temperature. Emotionally, it prevents us blowing 'hot and cold' in our relationships so that we maintain a balanced emotional temperature.

These multiple functions, that of the Heart Protector, the Three Heater and the Small Intestine, are all there to support and protect the Heart at their centre. If they function properly, the Heart will have sufficient time behind its protective mechanisms to assess its relationships and decide on how beneficial or not they are.

What happens if they function badly, and what can throw the Heart and its helpers out of balance in this way? To start with, a very vulnerable young baby may not live with parents or other adults who nurture its Heart properly. They may not be aware of the need to protect the child emotionally so as to help its little Heart Protector gain experience in a safe environment. They may give the baby and then the child confusing signals as to how to deal with relationships, perhaps by a mother screaming angrily at the father one minute and then showering him with kisses the next. A child is very sensitive to such changes in emotional temperature and its Three Heater function will struggle to maintain balance. If it is not advised wisely about which people it is safe for it to approach with its love, it will be understandably confused as its relationships develop.

When Fire's organs and functions do not do their work well, the Heart will function badly, ending a good relationship unwisely, lingering too long in a bad relationship, making friends of people we should be wary of, and turning away from people whose friendship would benefit us.

The Fire element: a case study

One of my Fire patients came for treatment because she suffered from recurring bouts of severe tonsillitis at different times of the year. She had also been told that she had the beginnings of what had been diagnosed as Raynaud's syndrome in her fingers. She had a tingling sensation down her middle finger, and the finger would go white and numb, even when it was not cold outside. She also told me that she could not cope with going out and meeting new people.

Her fear of people had started when she and her brother and sister had moved with her mother to a new town, leaving behind many good friends. Her first day at the new school had been very frightening, and she had been picked on and bullied as a new girl.

It turned out that the move had been caused by the break-up of her parents' marriage. Her mother had moved into the new home with a new boyfriend. Her father was very distressed by the break-up, and she had divided loyalties.

Her Fire element was not coping well with the difficulties the family pressures had created for her. Her Small Intestine (trying to sort the appropriate from the inappropriate) was confused by the conflicting demands. Her Three Heater was under stress from the constant emotional roller-coaster in the family (everybody blowing hot and cold all the time). Her Heart Protector was not doing a very good job of protecting the Heart because she felt devastated by what had happened.

Because the Fire element was under such stress, none of its organs or functions were working well. The cold fingers were a direct result of imbalance in the Three Heater. The tingling middle finger was exactly where the Heart Protector meridian runs (down the middle of the inner arm to the middle finger) and the lack of energy flowing along this meridian led to the tingling and the dead feeling in the finger.

Emotionally, her fear of making new friends was a result of weakness in her Heart Protector which felt that it could not cope with the many demands upon it made as she encountered all her new school mates, as well as trying to cope with her unhappiness about her parents.

She showed her imbalance in Fire by an absence of red in the face, by inappropriate laughter when talking about her troubles and by an exaggerated scorched smell. Her emotion showed an absence of joy when she talked about all the people nearest to her.

Treatment consisted in strengthening her Fire element by needling points on the Heart Protector and Three Heater meridians, where her greatest imbalance was.

As treatment helped her Fire element regain its balance, she reported changes at each visit. The first change I noticed was that she seemed altogether a little happier in herself. Her colour was now a much healthier pink, and she stopped the rather hysterical laughter which had been a way of stoking up her own Fire element.

Then she told me that she had made a new friend at school, and this friend was protecting her from the bullying. She had, in effect, found a Heart Protector in the outside world to shelter her. Gradually, her social life improved. She was asked out to a disco where she met some more friends. She began to look forward to going to school.

Things also improved at home. When she saw her father now, she did not feel so torn by his unhappiness and the conflict in loyalty was more tolerable.

The last things to improve were her physical symptoms, but by then she felt so much better in herself that these no longer concerned her as much as they did when she first came for treatment. The tingling in her middle finger (much helped by treatment on the Heart Protector meridian) gradually stopped, and the finger no longer went white and numb. The Three Heater was better able to keep the body's temperature even. Her attacks of tonsillitis, which had a lot to do with the Fire element's control over communication and speech, also grew less, as she felt more able to relate to other people.

One way of judging her improvement in general balance was by listening to how she talked about her relationship with her classmates and her family. From showing a great deal of hurt and vulnerability when she first came for treatment ('No-one wants to talk to me') she now said things like, 'The class is really very nice to me', or even 'I told the class bully to leave me alone', a sure sign that her Heart Protector was doing its work properly. As it grew stronger, it gave a protection to her former vulnerability, making it possible for her to enter safely into new relationships.

She was also better at judging who to be wary of and who to befriend so that her choices were more appropriate, and she no longer laid herself open to rejection as before. Within a few months of the start of treatment, she met her first boyfriend, and dealt well with all the difficulties sexual relationships bring in their wake – a sure sign of the Fire element's growing strength.

CHAPTER 19

THE EARTH ELEMENT

Season	Late summer
Time of day	07:00–11:00
Climate	Humidity
Organs	Stomach Spleen
Emotion	Sympathy
Colour	Yellow
Sound	Singing
Smell	Fragrant
Controls	Muscles and flesh

In old diagrams of the five element circle, Earth used to be in the centre, surrounded by the other four elements, as a mother is the centre of the family surrounded by her children. With Earth, we move into the world of the family and the home.

Thinking of Earth as the element of the centre helps us understand its function and also its needs. Earth pulls us towards it much like gravity pulls us to the ground below our feet. Like the earth on which we stand, the Earth element supports us, and provides us with the food which enables us to survive. It nourishes us like a mother her children.

Earth's two organs are the Stomach and the Spleen. The Stomach is the place where we digest the food and liquid we have taken in and convert it into nutrients for the body to use for all its purposes. In acupuncture terms, the Earth element not only nourishes our body, but it nourishes our mind and spirit as well, and has much to do with processing our thoughts. We know that we can 'churn things over' in our mind, and we can say that we 'can't swallow that', or 'can't stomach' something. Things 'stick in our gullet', too, if we do not like somebody's opinions. All these common expressions of speech recognize this deeper aspect of our Earth element.

Earth's season is late summer, our harvest time, after the deep heat of summer has passed and before the onset of the colder autumn days. Late summer is the time when the year turns from the lighter days towards the dark. In nature we see how the fruit on the trees weighs down the branches so that they are pulled down towards the earth. Late summer is the point where the year turns from the two outward yang seasons of spring and summer inwards to the two yin seasons of autumn and winter. The Earth element, too, holds a similar pivotal position among the elements. It can be said to look both ways, back to the summer which warmed its fruit, and forward to the autumn when its fruit has been plucked.

Like the hub at the centre of a wheel, Earth draws energy from the other elements on the outer rim of the wheel, and, in turn, gives back energy as it spirals on itself. It therefore both gives and receives, and has this dual function in all that it does. Before the mother can nourish her children, she must nourish herself to survive. Before the earth can yield fruit, it has itself to be fed with nutrients. The Stomach, too, can supply food to the other organs only when it has been fed itself.

This two-way movement is also there in its emotion, sympathy, which it can give as well as take, making it capable of being both generous and selfish at the same time. Sympathy is not a wide enough word to cover all the emotions Earth feels. It also understands and empathizes, feeling other people's pain as its own. This sensitivity can easily become too heavy a burden to bear, as it feels itself drained by the demands made upon it. Then it has to retreat into itself for a time to regain its strength and nourish itself before it can give of itself again.

It therefore has to temper its need to nourish others with a balanced assessment of when to stop giving before it finds it has nothing left to give. In balance, this makes it the most generous of elements, seeing to others' needs with real understanding. Out of balance, it will hold all it has selfishly to itself, unable to offer anything to others for fear that it will itself starve. This can turn a very unselfish element into a selfish element concerned only with itself.

Earth's function is to sustain the other elements, and it provides the foundation upon which they all rest. Stability is important to it and it cherishes having a firm base from which to work. It likes having its feet firmly on the ground. Any threat to its stability will disturb it, as though it is being shaken to its foundations. This is much like an earthquake rocking the ground beneath our feet. Aware that its stability may be threatened in this way, it clings more than any other element to a need for security. It makes of its home a place of great comfort and safety, and will be uneasy if it has to move house. 'As snug as a bug in a rug' is how Earth would like to be.

But wherever an element puts its greatest emphasis is also potentially the place of its greatest weakness. An element which places such great emphasis on nurturing itself and others will feel very deprived if this nurturing does not take place. Earth is the element above all which expects and demands a well-stocked larder. To be without food is for Earth as terrible as for Fire to be without love and for Wood to be unable to move.

Each element shows its imbalance in different ways, Wood by becoming frustrated at being hemmed in, Fire by becoming sad at being unable to give its love, and Earth by becoming unable to feed itself and others. An Earth mother out of balance might well be unable to feed her child at all. This may be one of the reasons why a mother cannot breastfeed her children. Alternatively, she may react by going to the other extreme and overfeeding her child, or being excessively worried if the child does not eat enough.

The tension which is always there in Earth between giving and taking away may tilt the scales to either side, making Earth people want to shower others with gifts they do not want, or grab all for themselves. Unable to take in food at an emotional level, too, they may stand as though before their own filled larder, unable to reach out to take the food. This may be what happens in cases of anorexia or bulimia where a person's Stomach craves food to excess, but has to vomit it out once it reaches its Stomach. The Earth element is here unable to decide whether to accept or reject the food its Stomach is offered.

Earth's colour is yellow, like the glow of a field of corn, or a sickly greyish-yellow when out of balance. Its voice has a singing quality to it, with the lilt of a lullaby in it. Its smell is called fragrant, a sweet, sometimes cloying, smell if its organs are out of balance.

The Earth element: a case study

A patient of mine came for treatment for digestive troubles and weight problems. She felt constantly bloated, craved sweet food and had very irregular periods. I diagnosed her as of the Earth element, whose organs are the Stomach and the Spleen.

She also told me that she had a very difficult relationship with her elder daughter, who was now 17. In the end, because of the constant disagreements between them, she had told her daughter to leave and move in with her father, my patient's ex-husband.

She always talked about this daughter with great anger, in marked contrast to the way in which she talked about her younger daughter from a second marriage. This child was the apple of her eye. What had gone so wrong in the first relationship, I wondered? Was it because the elder daughter was disturbed by the break-up of her parents' marriage? Why did I detect such a vein of bitterness whenever we touched on the subject of this daughter, which stretched back much further than the time of her parents' split-up?

The Earth element is the element of the mother, both of Mother Earth which provides us with food, and of the mother who bore us. Imbalances in the Earth element may often stem from difficult relationships with our mother and the degree to which she is capable of nurturing us adequately, both physically and emotionally. It turned out that my patient's own mother had had great problems in looking after her. She had been a very inadequate mother, often away from home, and demanding that her daughter look after herself and her younger sister, and do all the cooking and housework. When at home, her mother favoured the younger sister and denied my patient the attention every child craves from its mother.

In turn, as my patient became a mother herself, these difficult memories from her own childhood affected her relationship to her own first-born. It was as though she re-enacted the relationship she had had with her own mother in her own relationship to her elder daughter, replicating the denial of love and nurturing she had been given, and lavishing all her love on her second daughter, as her mother had done.

I viewed her problems with food as an inability to nourish herself properly because her mother had not nourished her when she needed it. This pointed to a very ambivalent attitude to food; she sometimes stuffed herself with chocolates, and at other times starved herself in order to lose weight.

Treatment was focused on strengthening the Earth element by needling points on the Stomach and Spleen meridians. As the Earth element within her became more balanced, her attitude changed both in relation to the food she ate and to providing food for others (feeding her children emotionally). She was surprised to find herself making contact with her elder daughter again, and enjoying both her daughters' company equally. After a few months of treatment, she arrived one day and said that she had asked her daughter to move back home. 'We seem to be getting on so well now.'

At a physical level, her periods became more regular. Her Stomach discomfort disappeared, and with it her craving for sweet food. Her weight stabilized, too, as her diet improved.

CHAPTER 20

THE METAL ELEMENT

Season	Autumn
Time of day	03:00–07:00
Climate	Dryness
Organs	Lung Large Intestine
Emotion	Grief
Colour	White
Sound	Weeping
Smell	Rotten
Controls	Skin and hair

When we have a good harvest, we use some of it as food, and put as much as we can of the remainder into store. Not every apple and pear, though, can be stored for our use. Some of them drop unpicked and uneaten to the ground, to be turned into compost for our gardens or trodden underfoot on the floor of the forest. But even the residue of the harvest bears a final fruit. It is here that the Metal element takes over from its mother, the Earth element, as autumn sets in. It is Metal's task to extract the last drops of goodness from the dying leaves, and deposit them in the soil as the trace elements which all growing things need to give them life.

If you look at a bottle of mineral water, you will be surprised at how many trace elements the water contains: calcium, magnesium, sodium, chloride and nitrate are but a few of the minerals within each bottle. They are invisible in the water, and yet without them nothing will grow. They are as essential for human growth as they are for the survival of all growing things in nature. They are like the essences we put in cakes to flavour them: a tiny drop of alcohol or vanilla essence will flavour the whole cake. The trace elements in the soil are distilled from the ripe fruits which the Earth element is there to offer, just as wine is distilled from ripe grapes. Much of this work is hidden and yet it is so essential to survival.

As well as the balance of minerals we find in the ground, Metal also controls the deposit of precious stones, such as diamonds, gold and silver, which human beings value so highly that a diamond the size of a walnut is worth a king's ransom, while a whole basket of walnuts is worth so little.

This is an image of how Metal adds quality to our life. Things become valuable through their rarity value and their purity. The purer the diamonds buried in the ground, the more valuable they are. The purer the trace elements we all depend upon, the greater their value. The Metal element spends its time assessing things on the basis of their purity value, discarding what is polluted and impure through the Large Intestine, our bowels.

Metal is preoccupied with assessing the true value of things, since what it extracts, though mere traces, must bear within it all the goodness the seeds of the next cycle need for their nourishment. It is a very discriminating, acutely sensitive element, aware of all the nuances of things and therefore, in its awareness, quick to take offence if others are less exacting. Its need of fine judgement makes it critical of shortcomings, both its own and those of others. This leads to a constant state of dissatisfaction, since it often feels that it has failed to live up to its own expectations and its high standards.

The Metal element's two organs are the Lung and the Large Intestine, one the organ of intake, giving us the breath of life, the other the organ of excretion, getting rid of all waste products. Our Lungs inhale pure air, sending this round the body in the blood. The Large Intestine, so closely linked to the Lung in Chinese medicine, is involved both in the exhalation of the waste from the air as we breathe out and in the excretion of solid waste products through the bowels.

To illustrate the close relationship of the two Metal organs, the last acupuncture point on the Large Intestine meridian is at the nose, where the Lung will breathe its next breath, not, as one might expect, in the lower part of the body near the physical bowel.

Purity and impurity are the two sides of the same coin, the pure breath the Lung needs depends on the exhalation beforehand of the waste products of that breath by the Large Intestine. That same tension between pure and impure is in all that the Metal element does.

Emotionally, it will tell us if something is an 'absolute waste of time' or 'rubbish', and this makes it by far the most discriminating element of all, constantly occupied with examining everything form the point of view of its value. 'Is this worth keeping, or shall I get rid of it?', it will ask itself.

And it has to do this very quickly, within the time needed to take one breath and the next. If we think of autumn, too, this is not a season which delays long, as summer and winter do. It is quickly over, the rich autumn colours on the trees fading almost before we have had time to admire them, as the sap withdraws from the leaves and they are left to wither and die.

One of the metal objects we use most commonly in everyday life is a knife or a pair of scissors. Both are there to cut things down to an appropriate size. Those with Metal as their constitutional element, too, can cut things down to size, including other people. Metal can be the most cutting of all elements, with a sharpness of tongue and wit which makes no bones about stating things the way it sees them and usually the way things actually are.

In balance, its self-criticism and criticism of others will be tempered by its acceptance of the burden of human frailties. Out of balance, they will be exaggerated into such mockery of others and of itself that it is paralyzed by feelings of such self-doubt and a mistrust of what it sees as the inadequacy of others that it loses a sense of the true value of things. It may then mistake quantity for quality, placing emphasis perhaps on the monetary value given to things by others rather than relying on its own discrimination.

Above all, we gain our self-respect if we put a proper value on ourselves and on what we do. If we do not have a true sense of such values, perhaps because the Metal element has never been strong enough to assess what is essential to take in and what to discard, we may rely on the judgement of others to guide us, accepting their values where we should rely on our own.

This might mean, for example, that we might place too great an emphasis on material things, wanting to emulate those with expensive cars or lucrative jobs because these are apparently ostentatious and visible signs of material success and thus a gauge of some value in the eyes of others. A true assessment would be to judge whether the person to whom the car, the money and the job belong are worth our respect, rather than taking the outer trappings for the inner person.

An imbalance in Metal can therefore lead us to misread what is valuable and worth keeping. It is as though we breathe in when we should breathe out, our Lungs not taking in the purity of the air and our Colon not getting rid of the waste. We can see how this might lead to breathing or bowel troubles, since the impurities the Metal element is meant to dispose of remain within us to pollute and unbalance us.

Metal's emotion is grief, its colour is white, its sound of voice weeping and its smell rotten, the smell of vegetation trodden underfoot on the forest floor in autumn. When in balance, this grief will show itself as a recognition of the inevitable advance of death at the end of all human life. When out of balance, it will prevent someone from letting go the feeling of grief about some loss suffered when this is appropriate. This can be an actual death, or it can be a loss of some kind, such as a friend leaving or failure in an exam, which can be seen as the loss of self-esteem. The Lung and the Colon will have difficulty coping with any major loss of this kind. The Colon is unable to let go of the grief, giving the Lung less space to take in new things. A person can be literally 'bunged up' in this way. (Constipation can be a sign of this inability to let go of the excess grief.)

The Metal element: a case study

John is a 17-year-old young man who came for treatment because he had had asthma since a child, and often had other bronchial problems. His chest was very tight and his breathing shallow. He had also suffered from severe constipation for most of his life. When asked about how his life was at the moment, he said that increasingly 'he couldn't cope with things'. He had just left school with sufficiently good A-levels to get into university, but he was not sure what or where he wanted to study. He wondered if he should take a year off to travel before going on to his studies. He was the youngest of three children, with two much older sisters. His father and mother were both highfliers, his father a consultant orthopaedic surgeon, his mother a barrister.

During the diagnosis, it became clear that the main reason why he could not cope was because of the great weight of expectation he felt his parents, particularly his father, had always laid upon him. He was the long-awaited only son, and there had been an unspoken expectation that he would follow his father into medicine. He felt throttled by the burden of his family's expectations. As he put it, 'I feel I can't breathe when I'm at home.'

I diagnosed him as of the Metal element, with the emphasis on the Lung meridian. He craved the respect of his much-respected father, but felt a failure because he was reluctant to follow in his father's footsteps. It was as though his father had cast a shadow over him all his life. In this shadow he felt stifled. The individual spark of life which is ignited the moment we take our first breath outside our mother's womb could not kindle a strong enough flame to enable him to move out from under his father's shadow to stand in his own sunlight.

He said that the only time he felt really relaxed was when his father was away. Then his mother's relationship to him would change, and he could feel for a short time that he was a person in his own right, with a sense of value in himself.

The Metal element, as we have seen, is the element which enables us to discern what is valuable and valueless in life. It helps us discriminate properly, and with this we gain a sense of our own identity. We see things as they are, ourselves included. This sense of identity, the ability to say 'I am who I am' despite what others want us to be, had been submerged in John beneath the stifling mantle of his father's dominant personality. He felt his father wanted him to be a son in his own image, denying him the right to be himself. There was a feeling of great emptiness in him, that emptiness which comes from a sense of loss of identity.

Because the Metal element was stifled in this way, John also suffered from problems affecting his Lungs. In my view, he was unable to take in, both the air he needed to breathe and emotional food. The reverse of this was the difficulty he experienced in letting go. The complementary organ to the Lungs is the Colon, the bowels. When our bowels function easily at a physical level, the body knows what it must eliminate to leave more space to take in further food. When the body is not sure what to eliminate, we tend towards constipation or diarrhoea, holding on too long to what we should let go or eliminating everything, the good nutrients as well as the waste products.

Since the Colon also has an effect on mind and spirit, its function is to clear waste products at these levels too. John's spirit was stifled, and his breathing congested. He had trouble in eliminating thoughts, and he could not clear his mind. He was obsessed with proving himself to his father, and yet he could not send off his university application form to study medicine. He did not know what he should let go of – his desire to please his father, or his desire to do his own thing.

Treatment consisted in treating acupuncture points on the Lung and Colon meridians. This helped to get rid of years of accumulated waste at all levels of body, mind and spirit. This in turn strengthened his sense of his own identity. The

Metal element in balance helps us gain a sense of who we really are. It is as though our Lungs are at last able to inhale air properly.

As his Metal element became stronger, he began to feel that he dared to 'do his own thing'. After a few months of treatment, he found that he could do without his inhaler for asthma, and his bowels had regulated themselves. One day he said that he had told his father that he did not want to study medicine, and to his surprise his father had made no objections. It seemed that the feeling that his father expected so much from him had partly been stoked by his own fears. John had felt that he should mould himself in his father's image. Once he was clear in himself about the direction he wanted to take – he decided to take a year off, and applied to study for an arts degree – his father accepted this readily, pleased to see his son so much happier in himself.

John now walked taller, surer of who he was, and his father started to respect him for this. Treatment had helped John to gain his own self-respect, and with that, that of his father. 'I now know who I am', he told me. This is Metal's gift to the other elements.

CHAPTER 21

THE WATER ELEMENT

Season	Winter
Time of day	15:00–19:00
Climate	Cold
Organs	Kidney Bladder
Emotion	Fear
Colour	Blue
Sound	Groaning
Smell	Putrid
Controls	Bones and marrow

Water is the alpha and omega of all the elements, their beginning and their end. It brings the cycle of the elements full circle. Indeed, that is its main function – to join things together. It creates the connection between things, the link between the end of the year and the start of the next year, as much as the link between the different cells in the body which allows them to function as a whole.

Water is the basic component of the universe. It is created from hydrogen atoms, the building blocks of the universe. These are the essential components from which matter and then the human being are formed. It is the dominant element in deepest space as it is inside each cell of our body. At least 80 per cent of our bodies, so apparently solid, are awash in water.

Water created us, and we were born in fluid, the placenta. Blood cannot flow without it. Tears cannot fall without it. No knee can bend without the synovial fluid to give it flexibility. No baby can survive without the water in its mother's milk.

Water is a cleansing, purifying element, both a baptismal blessing and the daily shower or bath we take to wash away the day's grime.

If we look down at the world from space, we see vast tracts of blue spreading over the surface where the oceans cover the land beneath. Nothing survives without water's blessing. No blade of grass or grain of rice, no animal or human, no fly or bird, can survive without water. We can survive without food for far longer than we can without water.

A leaf on the tree loses its shape once the water which creates its sap is drawn back to the roots in autumn. A fertile landscape can become the barren wastes of the American dustbowl or the Sahara by the slow withdrawal of water beneath it. Water can also be overpowering, creating torrents and floods out of gentle mountain streams, and, when frozen, pouring thundering avalanches down mountain sides. It has this ability to transform itself suddenly from the gentleness of a drop of dew into the awesome strength of a raging torrent. It can both give and take life. It can moisten our parched throats or drown us in its tides.

It can also change shape, and is the only element to do so. It can heap itself up into the great ice flows of the Arctic permafrost, it can be a babbling mountain stream, trickling over stones, or it can announce a train's arrival in a hiss of steam. This fluidity of form gives it an elusiveness no other element possesses. It has within it some of the mysteriousness of the ocean deep, a hidden quality hard to pin down and hard to grasp. Like the water whose name it bears, it melds easily with everything else, fitting in and going naturally 'with the flow'. A drop of water is almost invisible, evaporating with the first rays of the sun, and yet such little drops, when banded together, can form the implacable force which can cut deep into rock to carve out the Grand Canyon miles deep.

This power is in all Water people, and gives them their strength, making Water the strongest element of all. It creates the two organs, the Kidney and Bladder, and provides us with our reserves of energy and willpower. It is an ambitious element, knowing where it is going and determined to get there. It has little difficulty rising to the top as it finds its own level, and thus often achieves what it sets out to do.

Winter is its season, but, unlike hibernating animals, it does not settle down easily in its winter sleep, for winter brings with it its own terror, that of not surviving. Fear is water's emotion, the fear that lurks in all of us when we contemplate the hidden depth beneath us as we swim. Before the days of the freezer, we never knew in winter whether we had sufficient food to last the cold months until spring, and even now winter brings misery to many countries. For those trapped in snow, there is a very real fear they will not survive, just as those trapped by water itself will fear that they may drown. We have to struggle hard to survive for long in water, even though we may be strong swimmers. The treacherous currents and the effort it takes to keep our head above water all conspire to pull us down and drown us.

This fear of going under is present in Water's voice which has an apprehensive tremor in it, which we call a groaning voice. The colour the two Water organs send to the skin is a bluish black, which can be either translucent or an opaque colour.

Fear is not an emotion that animals must show in the wild, because a frightened animal attracts attention and will be attacked. In the same way, Water people will tend to hide their fear in an attempt to convince themselves and others that they are not frightened. The sense of fear may appear only in the way they appear as though frozen to the spot, like a rabbit caught in the headlights of a car, a form of paralysis which shows itself in rigidity, which is the opposite of the flow Water likes. It may also show its fear by sudden jerky movements or quick glances out of the corner of the eye to reassure itself that all is safe.

It is this reassurance that Water wants above all – the reassurance that it will survive come what may. Acupuncturists may find themselves speaking to a patient in a soothing tone and only become aware afterwards that they have been trying to allay the hidden fear they detect in their patient.

The Water element: a case study

A patient came to me for treatment for help with bad back pain and creaking knees. He sweated more than most people, and suffered from athlete's foot because of the dampness of his feet. He was a builder and had to lift very heavy weights in his work. I diagnosed his constitutional element as Water.

He found that he became very tired in the afternoon (Water time according to the Chinese clock) when his imbalance showed in its most exaggerated form. His back pain also increased steadily during the afternoon.

During our first meeting I noticed how taut to the touch his whole body was, as though his muscles were clenched. It seemed from what he said that his back trouble had started when he had gone into business on his own, and, as he put it, 'everything landed on my shoulders'. It was obvious that he was frightened that he had taken on too much responsibility. This fear had robbed him of the fluidity and ease which the Water element gives to us, tightening his back and making his knees creak. He needed a great deal of reassurance to convince him that things would improve, the reassurance that Water craves.

It turned out that he drank a good deal of tea and coffee, but very little water. Hot drinks tend to dehydrate us further, and we all need the lubrication water alone can provide. His Water element showed its lack of mobility and lubrication in the stiffness of the back and his creaking knees, and he needed more liquid intake than most people to offset this. The Bladder has a particular relationship to the back, and its meridians flow from the head down over the back to the legs, the back of the knees and the toes.

His acupuncture treatment consisted in needling points on the Kidney and Bladder meridians to strengthen the Water element. This had the effect of reducing the very real fear he had that his back trouble would force him to give up work. This in turn helped his body relax its tension so that his back pain eased and his knees moved more freely. The renewed strength in his back helped him to stand more upright and this enabled him to lift weights more smoothly without injuring himself.

I told him to drink more water and reduce his intake of tea and coffee. This improvement in fluid intake helped restore the fluid balance in his body, so that his feet were no longer so damp.

The general increase in the balance of the Water element ensured that he was able to adapt more easily to the demands of his work. He realized that he could no longer single-handedly do the work he had to do without injuring his back again, and decided to employ a younger assistant to do the heavy work. This extra help meant that the business was no longer so dependent on his health, and this allayed some of his fear that it might go under.

At the start of the treatment the image I had of him was of water that had been dammed and frozen over. After some treatment I saw him as water running easily between the banks of a river, smoothly avoiding the obstacles in its way. He now flowed, as all Water people like to do.

CHAPTER 22

How Elements Relate to Each Other

We have seen how the different constitutional types we call by the names of the elements have different needs and different responses to the demands of life. We are now going to look at how we accommodate these differing needs and responses to those of the people around us. We will see how our knowledge of the different elements helps us understand our relationships with other people better.

Our interactions with other people start from our earliest days, initially with our mothers, fathers and families. As we grow older, they spread out to encounters with people further afield, our friends, partners and colleagues. Throughout all this, we have to learn to make adjustments so that we can live easily with people who differ in their constitutional make-up from ourselves.

It is useful to take a moment to think of those closest to us. We have no choice in selecting our family, but we can and do choose friends and partners. If we look carefully at these, we will find that we have a surprising capacity to move towards people who are different from us and stimulate us in some way. It is as though their very difference from ourselves attracts us to them. Seen from the point of view of the elements, it would appear that we enjoy the challenges different elements give to such encounters. I like to think this is humanity's way of extending its variety as a species, much like a horticulturalist will graft different varieties of plants on to one another to increase the stock available.

You may be surprised how varied your circle of friends is, each friend probably giving you something different. Perhaps one is sympathetic to your troubles, the other makes you laugh, and yet another pushes you to do things you didn't know you could do. Each one of them in their own way will have something different to offer you.

The same is true of our choice of partners. As with friends, the partners we choose enrich our lives, if we choose wisely, or diminish our lives, if we choose unwisely. And when our choices are made to stimulate us and give our lives variety, we often find that we choose people whose constitutional element differs from ours.

How we approach other people will have been shaped by our early family relationships and by the extent to which these have been harmonious and fulfilling. Our early life may have allowed us to blossom as a unique individual, as we should, or it may have stunted our emotional growth, so that we have had to learn to hide our needs.

The more we are encouraged to be ourselves as a child, the more the energy of our elements will flow healthily round our bodies, minds and spirits. When this is so, we use this good energy in our encounters with other people so that our judgement is sound and we see those we meet through eyes unclouded by our own problems. Such a state of balance will enable us to choose partners and friends from amongst those people who are most suited to satisfy our needs, and stimulate us to greater development.

As we have seen, the nature of these needs and of our potential is deeply associated with those of our constitutional element. Those who are of the Water element, and require some degree of security and certainty in their life, may well look to people who provide such security. Conversely, if the Water element is out of balance, they may look to relationships in which there is some degree of risk (Water's emotion, fear out of balance, being attracted to situations in which danger is present).

In balance, we will all be looking for relationships which enhance us. In element terms, this will mean that these relationships will strengthen our constitutional element, allowing it room to expand and develop.

In an ideal world, if all of us were balanced human beings, our relationships with others would look like this:

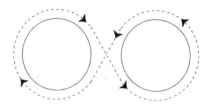

Each of us would remain whole (all the elements flowing in a beautiful circle within us), whilst allowing a unifying, creative flow to envelop the two of us. We are joined together within this relationship, but remain ourselves.

The reality of human life, with its stresses, often distorts this picture. We may not be a beautiful whole, and the people we encounter may also have their own problems. The encounter between us will then be very different, and look more like this:

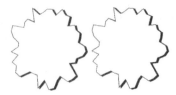

Here the relationship between the two of us does not flow easily, as our jagged edges tear at each other. In extreme cases, they tear us apart (messy divorces, alienation from our parents or our children). In less extreme cases, we may learn to accommodate other people's jagged edges, provided they are prepared, in their turn, to accommodate ours. With time, and with goodwill and perseverance on both sides, the jagged edges may be smoothed away into something more closely resembling a circle. This is what occurs when partnerships go through a rocky passage, and then strengthen themselves, or when we argue with a friend and then mutually agree to be more tolerant of each other.

Such jagged edges, appearing in a parent, have a very crippling effect on children, since a parent's unsatisfied needs will place unreasonable demands upon the growing child.

It is no wonder that the potential for difficult relationships is very great in such a complex world. And this makes it all the more heartening to discover that by recognizing the needs of the different elements we become much more tolerant. If we understand a little why other people are different from us, we will not find such differences threatening, and will allow other people the space to be themselves.

Treatment gradually smoothes our jagged edges so that they no longer tear at our friends and partners. People coming for acupuncture treatment often find that, as they become stronger, the difficulties they are experiencing in their relationships of all kinds (home, friends, at work) grow less, as they learn to understand themselves and others better. With this understanding comes a better appreciation of what others need, and thus more tolerance and less scope for conflict.

CHAPTER 23

ACUPUNCTURE AND WESTERN MEDICINE

You will have begun to understand from what you have read so far that Chinese medicine's approach to health and ill-health and its way of diagnosing and treating are very different from those of Western medicine. Increasingly, however, we are seeing that the two different systems of medicine are learning to respect and live with each other.

This is very important for the future of health-care in the West, as the costs of drug therapy and surgical intervention continue to rise so steeply. Because acupuncture is so cost effective, it is very attractive to those concerned with the future of health-care. Its side-effects, if any, are minimal and its success rate is high.

Acupuncture also emphasizes the importance of self-help as part of treatment, involving patients in their own treatment and encouraging them to take control of their own health. Diagnosis and treatment are cooperative efforts between patient and practitioner, and their close relationship is one of the reasons for acupuncture's increasing popularity.

The Western medical world is increasingly interested in what acupuncture can do. Its success in pain relief and in mitigating the side-effects of treatments such as chemotherapy or radiotherapy is well documented. Nurses now use it to help in childbirth.

But where acupuncture is making important inroads is in that wide and ever-growing range of illnesses for which Western medicine has no cure, and sometimes even no name, the 'non-specific' illnesses at which doctors shake their heads. In acupuncture terms, these are not seen as puzzling, but as a sign of imbalance in the energy of one or other element.

Often, too, treatment at a sufficiently early stage will prevent those illnesses which start as mild discomfort from turning into the major illnesses which crowd Western hospitals. Acupuncture's role as preventive medicine is not recognized by conventional medicine or by the lay public as fully as it be should be, but it will be here that I predict the greatest advances will be made. It is here, too, where acupuncture's contribution to the health of the population will most clearly be shown and recognized.

The growing partnership between acupuncture and its Western counterpart will become even stronger as acupuncture takes its place in mainstream medicine in the West.

INDEX